PRAISE FOR FATHERS AT BIRTH:

"Rose St. John has combined her immense amount of experience with assisting and teaching couples into a practical, no-nonsense, down-to-earth guide for fathers. Her recommendations for breathing, focusing, and coping are techniques that not only apply to labor and birth but are skills that will impact fathers and mothers for a lifetime. I am excited to see such a complete compendium directed at fathers, to know that it will help so many women have better and more pleasurable birth experiences."

—*Barbara Harper, RN, CLD, CCE, author of Gentle Birth Choices and Director of Waterbirth International*

"Fathers at Birth has sage advice for one and all. I am certainly recommending this book in my practice as a doula."

—*Patricia Woodbury, Birth/Postpartum Doula and Certified Happiest Baby Educator.*

"I congratulate Rose on the manifestation of this very meaningful, extremely helpful birthing guide for fathers to be. As a labor and delivery nurse I experience on a daily basis how scary and overwhelming labor can be for unprepared partners. The significant other often feels helpless and unequipped to adequately support his laboring loved one. By reading this book he will prepare himself for the birth experience, both by gaining knowledge about the birthing process as well acquiring a big bag of practical tools and helpful strategies for supporting his partner (and himself!) during labor.

"Not only will this greatly reduce his stress and empower him, it will support both his and his partner's ability to cope with the challenges of labor and ultimately enhance their birth experiences. I highly recommend this easy-to-read birthing book for any father-to-be, whether it is his first or subsequent child, and whether the couple chooses to birth their baby at home, at a birthing center, or in a hospital setting."

—*Tina Zeeberg, RN, BSN, labor and delivery nurse*

"My husband and I have been drawn closer as we have read this book and used both its principles and its practical tasks to prepare for the birth of our baby. I was drawn in and retained the information in a way that surprised me. I highly recommend this book and also suggest reading it as a couple.

—*Liana Mangan, Independent Consultant, District Manager, Arbonne International*

"I am excited about the fresh perspective that Rose has shown about my role as the father in this birth experience. To [learn] both the things that I can do and the boundaries beyond which not to step is immensely helpful. Rose [illustrates] how I can meaningfully contribute and help maximize our experience in this anticipated event.

—*Ryan W. Mangan, (husband of Liana Mangan) Weyerhaeuser Engineering Services*

D0424516

FATHERS AT BIRTH

Your Role in Bringing Your Child into the World

by

Rose St. John

ACKNOWLEDGMENTS

I owe a special debt of gratitude to Laurie Ludes, the talented and exquisite photographer of this book; Matt and Jeanette Swafford, who graciously agreed to be photographed and generously gave of their time; Catherine Parisi, the excellent midwife and director of the Connecticut Childbirth & Women's Center who opened doors and in every respect supported my work; Cherry Brandstater, MD, who contributed her expertise; publisher and editor Linda Meyer and publicist Allison Collins at Ink & Paper Group, LLC; book designer Alan Dubinsky; and illustrator Tyler Ownings who guided me with their expertise and oversaw the packaging, publicity, and publication of this book; my teachers who generously shared their expertise and to whom I am indebted; my clients, who made this work possible and taught me as much as I taught them; and the men for whom this book is written.

My special thanks and love go to my children, who helped me open to the possibilities available during labor and birth, and most of all to my husband, who patiently encouraged me through the whole process of birthing this book.

ABOUT THE AUTHOR

Rose St. John has spent the past twenty-five years, logging over 5,000 hours teaching and guiding couples through pregnancy and birth.

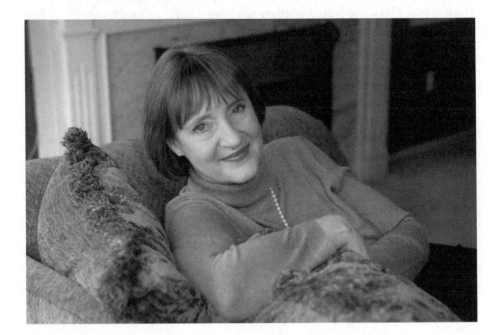

CONTENTS

PART ONE
GAINING A PERSPECTIVE
DEFINING YOUR ROLE

PART TWO
GETTING READY
THE PREPARATION

PART THREE
PREPARATION PRACTICES

PART FOUR
LABOR AND BIRTH

EPILOGUE
GOING HOME
THE FIRST FORTY DAYS AND BEYOND

APPENDICES
QUICK TIPS FOR LABOR

VIII

FOREWORD

Only in the last forty or fifty years have women's voices been heard as they express their desires to share their experiences with their families, and only in the last twenty-five to thirty years have they been truly listened to.

Much has been written about the emotional and physical aspects of birth with regard to mothers and newborns, but not much exists for fathers.

Rose St. John's book, *Fathers at Birth: Your Role in Bringing Your Child into the World*, delves into the father's role not only as a "birth coach," but as a physical, spiritual, and emotional guide for his partner during pregnancy, birth, and beyond. Ms. St. John clearly outlines the enormous relational benefit the father may derive from being a rock of support through the entire process.

Chapter by chapter, she provides detailed instruction on the inner workings of the pregnancy and the birth process. The aid she provides is heartening as she looks inside the mind of the laboring woman and shows the father why his role is so important.

The techniques for the father to use to guide and protect his partner are quite clear and functional. Her lessons are easy to understand, and appear fun for both mother and father. The book focuses on making the father as involved and informed as possible. He receives information on how to be the supportive cornerstone of the team while the mother is so vulnerable in labor. Help on choosing care providers, options for birth (including facilities, positions, and the use of water), and then instructions for care in the days following birth are all clear, and most importantly, helpful!

I applaud Ms. St. John on her enormous effort; she has taken a lifetime of experiences as a mother, doula, yoga instructor, birth coach, and birthing woman, and rolled them into a clear, easy-to-read guide for the most important attendant at the birth: THE FATHER.

Congratulations!

—Catherine/Cathi Parisi, CNM, Director of Connecticut Childbirth and Women's Center

THE INFAMOUS
TAXICAB DELIVERY STORY

A taxicab driver is transporting his pregnant and groaning passenger to the hospital when he hears the desperate, pressing words: *The baby's coming!* The driver's first reaction is: *No way, lady. Not in my cab.* But what he says is: *Hang on. We'll be there soon.*

Next he hears the woman vigorously panting and shrieking in his backseat. Although he is bewildered, the urgency of the unavoidable reality forces him to pull off the road. On the spot, the taxicab driver switches modes. He shifts out of his denial and reluctance to participate, and shows up. He morphs into a willing attendant, ready to do whatever he can.

With no prior experience and no training, he attends and assists the woman while she births her baby. Telling the new mother what a great job she did and what a beautiful baby she has, he places the babe in the new mother's arms. The woman is so grateful, she asks him his name, and announces she is naming the baby after him. Then the taxicab driver, with renewed perspective and wonder, continues the drive to the hospital.

So why am I telling this story? Everyone has heard a version of it, and no one wants to consider a taxi delivery as an option for birth. But what does it have to do with you, a father-to-be?

Just like the driver, an expectant father is already equipped to attend his partner during childbirth; the secret is switching modes. The driver has to shift out of his angst and habitual way of thinking so he can see and respond to the situation as it is. Not how he wants it to be. He has to show up and *play it as it lays.*

In this story, the driver and the woman discover their capacity beyond the edge. While neither wants a taxi delivery, when push comes to shove, they immerse themselves, and they succeed. Often the biggest challenge we face is the challenge of getting out of our own way, so we can see and respond without an agenda—without doubt, anxiety, or desire superimposed over the situation. When we release tension in the body, let the breath flow, and focus the mind, we are free to draw what we need from our innate resources, and respond to the situation at hand.

Discovering we have greater potential than we realize is one of the irrevocable truths of an immersion event like birth.

PART ONE

Gaining a Perspective: Defining Your Role

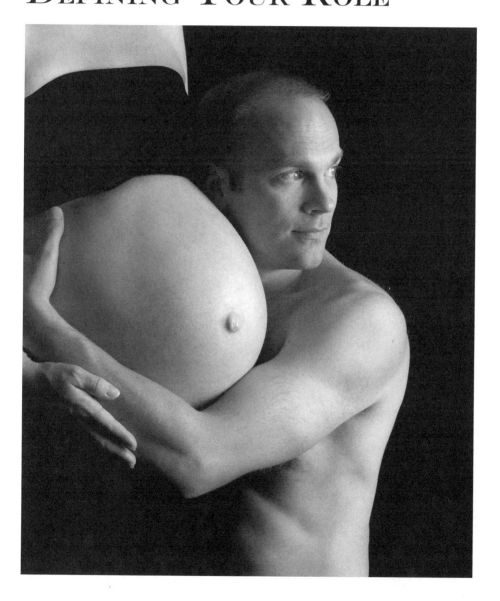

CHAPTER 1
YOUR PRESENCE MAKES A DIFFERENCE

THE JOURNEY

Imagine you are required to take a journey into an uncharted frontier, one that will tax you to your max, push you beyond known boundaries, and require you to persevere through the unknown, until you accomplish your mission. On this expedition, you must chart your own course. No one else can do it for you. But you can take a companion with you.

What type of companion would you choose? Would you choose someone who is distracted, someone who sidetracks and disturbs you? Or would you prefer someone who is focused, someone who has the skills to help you find your way and ease you over rough terrain? You'd choose the latter, of course. Similarly, this is the type of companion your partner wants you to be as she finds her path through labor.

During labor, your partner is absorbed in a challenging passage that demands her all. She must continue until the journey is complete, and she does not have the option or the luxury of turning back. Most men want to assist their partners through the demanding terrain of labor and birth, and they want the satisfaction of knowing they did the best job they could.

Jake said it like this: *I want my wife to have the best birth possible, and I want to know how to help her do that.*

If you want to know what a laboring woman needs from her partner and how to meet those needs, this book is for you. Simply by your attentive and responsive companionship, you influence the course your partner takes and how the journey unfolds. This handbook equips you with the wisdom and tools you need to be a skilled companion while you travel together through the uncharted frontier of labor and birth.

CHAPTER 1

MEN, LOVERS, AND FATHERS

No one other than the mother is more personally and profoundly affected by the baby's birth than you are. As the mother's lover and the baby's father, you are connected to them like no other. Your role—to provide stability and refuge—is unique to you. Most men want to do this. But many are uncertain how to offer genuine support during labor and birth. They especially don't want to do anything to get in the way or hinder the process.

Michael, a father expecting his second child, said: *At our first birth, I had no idea how important it was to my wife for me to know how to support her. There is so much I wish I had known. A man needs to be able to wrap his mind around what he needs to do. We attended classes, but I didn't get what I needed to know. I really want to be there for her during our second birth.*

Luke, a father expecting a second child, told me: *Men are pretty straightforward. If you just show me what needs to be done, give me some basic instruction, and get out of my way, I can do it.* In the heat of labor, I have witnessed the truth of Luke's statement. When a man knows how to be attentive and responsive, the mother breathes easier and her position softens because she knows her partner is with her.

Whether you are a seasoned or first-time father-to-be, this book will help you identify and refine the skills that matter most. I am excited to share with you what I have practiced for twenty-five years. I know this book will alter how you perceive and respond to your partner's labor. After reading it, you will have a clear understanding of a man's role during labor and birth.

You will learn simple concepts and practices that prepare you. You will understand why your stability is so important to your partner, and you will know how to recoup it if you lose it. You will know how to touch and talk to a laboring woman. You will learn tested strategies that work in the heat of labor to support you both. And you will acquire the insight and skills you need to be a companion who makes a genuine difference in labor and birth.

The practices and strategies in this book have been tried and refined in the fire over the years I spent teaching prenatal and postnatal yoga, couples' birth preparation classes, and attending my clients' births. They are also personal—my husband and I have used these same practices and strategies in the births of our children. What I teach has made a striking and significant difference for my clients' births. And it can make a significant difference for you and your partner in your birth experience.

MY BACKGROUND AND WHY IT MATTERS

Through the birth of my first child, I discovered birth was a richer and vaster experience than I had anticipated. My first birth was hugely challenging, but hugely rewarding. Even though I had planned to go though labor without drugs, I hit a point where I couldn't go on. However, labor was moving powerfully and swiftly, and by the time the nurse came in, drugs in hand, I had to push.

I narrowly escaped having drugs in my first labor. Having full sensation to push out my baby was profoundly satisfying and so was discovering that my body instinctively knew what to do and had the strength and wisdom to guide me through it. I just needed to get out of my own way enough to follow my body's lead.

Within three months of my first birth, I started practicing yoga under the guidance of Swami Rama, an accomplished yogi and founder of the Himalayan International Institute of Yoga Science and Philosophy. He instructed me in breathing (pranayama), hatha yoga, relaxation, meditation, spirituality, and more. His presence and teachings were riveting, and the results were deep and redirecting.

I taught yoga at a branch center of the Himalayan Institute, and attended many of the trainings held at various centers, and in India. I learned from the expert staff of doctors and psychologists who taught at the Himalayan Institute, as well as from teachers in other traditions. I learned about anatomy and physiology, diet and nutrition, homeopathy, biofeedback, wellness, psychology, philosophy, scriptures (sacred writings), meditation, and more. I began to use what I was learning and practicing to work with women and couples, helping them to prepare for labor and birth, and also attending the births. Eventually, I worked in a birthing center, as well as yoga studios, and doctors' offices. As a registered yoga teacher (E-RYT 500), I train and certify yoga teachers in prenatal, birthing, and postnatal yoga, and designed a birthing method based on meditation principles.

What I taught my clients made a dramatic impact in their births, and it made a dramatic difference for my husband and me in our subsequent two births. It completely altered how I experienced labor, and decreased anxiety and pain. I managed the challenge of waves and felt undisturbed and cradled in love during my second labor. It was a mystical experience. By my third birth, I was totally, consciously immersed in the waves of labor, and I felt pressure, but no pain. It was an experience of grace.

This is why I work with others going through pregnancy and birth. I know, from my own experience, the value of what I teach. I have seen the difference it makes in my clients' births, in their transitions after birth, and in their relationships. Since I believe the family is the bedrock of society, I offer this work to the men who attend their partners during labor and birth.

THE UNIQUE CONTRIBUTION OF MEN

Since you know your partner intimately, the unique contribution that only you, the father of her baby, can make to labor and birth cannot be overlooked. Katie expressed this need to have her partner with her: *I needed to know my husband—the other half of this baby who was being born—was with me. And I needed to know I wasn't doing this alone.*

Sharing the challenge of labor and the miracle of birth deepens the level of respect and regard a couple has for one another. Brenda described the shift that occurred in their relationship: *My husband's attendance at our birth was absolutely critical. It changed the whole dynamic of our relationship. Our connection increased exponentially. His commitment to me felt like a force. I knew he was there for me.*

Even though a woman prepares for labor—without support—it is not always easy for her to practice what she knows. This is why your preparation and support is so important to her. Manny commented on how preparation made a difference for him: *It was extraordinary to have the confidence to go in there knowing I had the tools I needed. If something didn't work, there was no crisis because I knew I had another tool I could use. That's when I realized how important the preparation work had been.*

Holly shared how her husband made the crucial difference: *I can't imagine what labor would have been if my husband hadn't been with me. He was my anchor. He kept me grounded. Because of him, I got through labor without drugs.*

Joseph, who attended his partner's birth, shared: *Men like to take action. But during labor, it's more about being in the moment with your partner and being watchful and supportive. For me, labor was an observance, a vigil. I had to show up and keep showing up.*

You profoundly influence your partner and how she navigates through labor. As a vigilant witness, your presence is as solid as a rock and as light as a feather, which gives your partner tremendous refuge and freedom. Your vigil, surprisingly, has the power to alter how labor and birth unfold. Proof of this is cited in quantum theory, which describes a subtle interconnectedness between all matter; and observation may alter the interconnectedness. Our attentive presence has the power to alter the outcome of an event.

Because the man's role can make such a critical difference, it is important men have access to the preparatory attention they need to fulfill their roles. I have written this book specifically for men, so they have access to the concepts, practices, and tools they need to be the best birth companion possible.

If families are to remain strong, men and their roles as partners, husbands, protectors, and fathers cannot be considered dispensable or superfluous. Both partners are diminished when the value of a man's contribution is marginalized, minimized, or not acknowledged. When the man's vital role during labor and birth is understood, both men and women are empowered.

THE PRACTICAL AND THE TRANSCENDENT

I have written this book with two goals in mind. The first is to share my experiences, to teach you practical skills and give you tools that work. This book presents the concepts, clearcut instructions, and hands-on practices you need to be a stable and adept companion, able to provide support. My target is for you to have the skills you need to be a strong birth partner, so you have the freedom to respond with confidence while you contribute to the celebrated birth of your child.

The second goal is to share my perspective on the transcendent, sacred aspect of birth. Even though birth is an everyday, everywhere occurrence, the birth of your child is an extraordinary day in your life. Birth draws us close to the mystery. Whenever we encounter the mystery, we know it. We are altered by it. But it is a rare day we participate directly with it. I want you to have the freedom to immerse yourself in the event, taking in the richness with more joy.

The purpose behind both these goals is for you to have the satisfaction of knowing you did the best job you could to fulfill you and your partner's desire to have the most rewarding birth possible.

CHAPTER 2

YOUR ROLE: THE MOUNTAIN AND THE WARRIOR

BE THE MOUNTAIN

A mountain's presence is its power. It is rock-solid. Silent. Still. Majestic. Upright. Massively and indisputably present—always there. Yet it doesn't do anything. It simply stands. Masculine energy is like a mountain's stability. Seeing yourself as the mountain gives you a picture of the most important skills you need to be a partner who makes a concrete difference at labor and birth.

A mountain doesn't need to do anything for its power to be apparent. If you push against a mountain, it does not collapse, get agitated, or try to control the situation. It remains unperturbed and steadfast. By being the mountain, you maintain your vigil and offer your partner the strength of your stable presence. This is the type of power Clair, one of my clients, experienced from her partner: *The thing that helped me most in labor was having my husband there, because I knew I wasn't alone. Somehow, his presence gave me a sense of safety. It made me feel like it was safe to open and bring this baby into the world.*

Do not underestimate the power of your stable presence. It helps your partner feel safe, which in turn helps her open with less resistance as she labors and births your baby.

MOUNTAIN PRESENCE AND RESERVE ENERGY

In a vital partner relationship, masculine energy flows from the male body into the female body. If you think about sexual intercourse, you have a picture of how masculine energy flows into the feminine body. During intercourse, the man's energy—his seed and potential—flows into the woman's body. The female body receives, contains, recreates, and redistributes the energy.

From this perspective, the two bodies are one body. Your partner draws from the reserve pool of your masculine energy and uses it to stabilize herself. Masculine power lies in the steadfast presence of the mountain as well as in the concentrated, wise potential of the seed.

9

When combined with feminine power, it breaks out and explodes into new life, a new order.

Since your masculine energy is available on many levels, your mere attentive presence allows your partner to draw from it. Here is Miranda's comment about her partner's concentrated potential: *My husband was pretty quiet during labor, but I could feel all this love coming from him. I remember thinking, 'I didn't know he loved me so much.' It helped me to get into this space where I could deal with labor.*

Olga shared: *My husband's presence as the mountain was very real to me. Very tangible. Incredibly important. Others in the room could be busy doing whatever, but I needed my husband to be my rock and stay physically close and present. Being able to hear him breathe between contractions calmed me down and helped me rest.* Don't dismiss the value of what you have to give simply by being there.

No one else can birth the baby for the mother. But being alongside her with your stable presence is a powerful component of your partner's sense of well-being. It provides a firm base for her to rely on as she finds her path through labor—a path she must find for herself. Sean shared: *I was struck by how just being there and staying focused was about 90 percent of it. Just being stable and not wandering away, or vacating, or thinking I wasn't important. It was amazing, absolutely amazing.*

It is not about what you say or do in labor. It is more about who you are. Be the mountain.

THE WATER

While masculine energy is like a mountain, feminine energy is like water. Because water is a fluid force, it changes quickly, without warning. It can surge and thrash one moment, and be reflective and calm the next. Your partner may exhibit water-like behavior during labor, but do not be misled. Flowing water carves through rock and surging water breaks through an impasse.

Charles expressed how the concept of mountain-and-water-energy helped him respond to his partner during labor: *My wife thrashed and pulled and pushed, and then she would just collapse and rest. I had this image of a woman thrashing and subsiding like water flowing down a mountain. That image was critical because it helped me stay calm and hold the space while she thrashed. It kept me from getting mental about it or stepping in to try to fix it.* When you hold the space like a mountain, your partner's water energy is free to find its course.

Labor and birth use assertive and authoritative power that arises in wave rhythms, like the surf of the ocean. The surging and primal energy of birthing takes many couples by surprise. As Joel explained, it can be quite astonishing: *I was surprised by how forceful and aggressive labor was. A human being gets pushed out, one wave at a time, from inside the person you care about. Birthing is a force to be reckoned with.*

The force of birthing is the embodiment of new life, which exposes the core of feminine power. Neither you nor your partner controls this force. Go with it and let it surge and flow. The mountain augments the flow of water.

BE THE WARRIOR

Along with being steadfast like a mountain, you also need to be alert and responsive like a warrior. A warrior gathers all his energy into one stream, one focus, so he can perceive and respond to the environment of battle. He must remain attentive and available (in vigil), but he must also be prepared to serve and protect.

Seeing yourself as a warrior gives you a picture of the most important skills you need to respond to your partner and protect her. A laboring woman is vulnerable and needs to be protected. As a matter of fact, if the mother does not feel protected, her labor can shut down. Holly, my client, explained it well: *In labor, I am in a much more vulnerable state, and not just physically. My perceptual net is more expanded. I am more sensitive to how my husband is doing. And I am more sensitive to everything going on around me. I need to tune out distractions and concentrate. I need more protection, and I need my husband to provide a buffer for me.*

Your warrior presence provides a buffer of protection that liberates your partner from extraneous concerns. This is a great gift to your partner as it frees her to use her energy exclusively to open and give birth.

THE MARK OF A WARRIOR: UNITE YOUR ENERGIES

One way you provide a buffer for your partner is to operate as a warrior does, from a position of power. To do so, you need to unite your energies. Imagine being a charioteer traveling with a team of untrained horses running in random directions. The charioteer must use tremendous energy to manage the horses while he journeys. He risks getting sidetracked, distracted, agitated, exhausted, and lost.

CHAPTER 2

Now imagine traveling to a destination as a charioteer who directs trained horses to move in ordered unison. He travels in the direction he chooses to go, and has more focus, ease, and power as he travels. This is how the application of uniting your energies works. When your energies are united, you are focused, responsive, and powerful like a warrior. This makes you vigilant in the heat of labor.

Each of us consists of several levels that are present in the here and now. We have a physical body, a breathing body, a mental body, an emotional body, an individual soul, and the pervading absolute that sustains and is beyond all those levels. When these levels are dissipated and fragmented, we disturb others and ourselves. When these levels are integrated and united, we have power and purpose. Our elevated sense of purpose elevates the purpose of those around us, gives them more power, and influences how situations unfold.

If you observe the body, you see three clearly defined sources of power protected by bone—head, chest, and pelvis. When these three sources of power are aligned, you draw on the strength of each of them to make you a formidable warrior. You draw from the rational strength of the head to make decisions. You draw from the instinctive strength of the gut to help you respond on the spot. You draw from the intuitive strength of the heart and offer the most inspiring force of all—love—devotion and commitment.

When your sources of strength are integrated, you have access to your power, which makes you a vigilant warrior, offering the mother tremendous protection, support, refuge, and strength.

BE CENTERED

Being centered is a characteristic the mountain and the warrior share. When you are centered, you are calm and alert; thus you can observe and respond to the mother's changing needs. When we tense up, it is often because we realize we are not in control. We do not know what to do, so we armor ourselves to maintain a semblance of order. This sometimes works as a short-term reaction. However, as a long-term approach in the vigil of labor, tension drains you and causes you to miss the mark.

Think of the difference between traveling with trained horses as opposed to being sidetracked by untrained horses. If your energies are dissipated and disconnected, the untrained horses sidetrack both you and the mother. If you are centered, you both have the advantage of traveling with trained horses. You must center your whole self, be-cause you cannot be an effective birth companion if:

- Your body is out of alignment, tense, and uncomfortable
- Your breath is haphazard and restricted
- Your emotions are vacillating and pulling you in different directions
- Your mind is confused, distracted, anxious, or in turmoil

If you are distracted or disturbed, you distract and disturb your partner. If you are centered, it helps the mother to center, which greatly reduces anxiety and pain. Take refuge in the knowledge that the one element your partner needs is your centered, attentive pres-ence. Your attentive presence is grounded in relaxation. And relax-ation is grounded in alignment and fluid breathing. To help you be-come skilled in the art of centering, I offer the following three-step, one-minute centering practice.

THE BASIC ONE-MINUTE CENTERING PRACTICE

On the spot, in less than a minute, you can coordinate and integrate the many facets of your being into a united force. By using the three-step, one-minute centering practice, you can quickly and effectively:

- Align and relax your body
- Allow the breath to flow and synchronize
- Focus your mind and direct your attention

You do this by asking and responding to three important questions: How am I using my body? How am I using my breath? How am I us-ing my mind?

1. HOW AM I USING MY BODY?

Observe your body. Turn your attention into your body and occupy the space your body occupies. Drop your armor. Release and relax your body to the best of your ability on the spot. Align and balance the three body weights—pelvis, chest, and head. Scan your body and give it whatever additional support it needs to be comfortable.

Alignment and relaxation conserve energy and help you remain at ease. Misalignment puts unnecessary pressure on your nerves, or-gans, and joints, which increases tension and stress. Alignment and relaxation have a subtle, yet powerful influence on how you perceive yourself, how you respond to a situation, how people respond to you, and how each situation unfolds.

2. HOW AM I USING MY BREATH?

Observe your breath. Feel the flow of breath in your nostrils. Let your forehead be smooth, and soften your eyes. Release restrictions, pauses, and noises in the breath, and let it be fluid and rhythmic. Don't force or control the breath. Think of the rhythm of ocean surf, and allow your breath to flow in and out. Since breath is the link between body and mind, breath has the power to calm the body and focus the mind. Your nervous system is intimately connected to breath and how you breathe affects how your entire system operates.

3. HOW AM I USING MY MIND?

Observe your thoughts. Release random thoughts, critical comments, doubts, worries, and mind noise. Then focus the mind on the situation. Focusing the mind is ongoing and radically alters how you perceive and respond. It gives you the freedom to respond to a situation instead of reacting out of habit.

Mind has the capacity to concentrate, discern, and receive revelation. It is advocate, problem solver, and guide. But mind is a double-edged sword. It can play the role of a wolf that devours you or a trickster that deceives you. Mind is subtle and can travel anywhere, but body remains limited in time and space. Let your mind occupy your body and breath. Then focus it on the situation at hand. Distracting thoughts will continue to flow. Observe and release them.

The three-step, one-minute centering practice is the main one you will use to maintain your labor vigil. It lets you observe and respond to your partner's changing needs. Use it whenever you need assistance or guidance. In less than a minute, you can align and relax the body, let the breath flow, and focus your mind on the situation at hand. Begin using it now. You have begun the process of becoming the mountain and the warrior your partner needs you to be.

CHAPTER 3
How To Communicate with a Laboring Woman

MEN'S AND WOMEN'S DIFFERING ANXIETIES

Five men from my birth preparation classes communicated their observations on the differences between men and women, and shared some of their anxieties about labor. Here are their comments:

Women's bodies are so mysterious. Their bodies can do so much. Their flow is tied to the moon and the waters. I don't understand it, but I am so influenced by it. Men don't have that.

Women are so different from men. I can't believe the changes in my wife's body. I just look at her and go, "Whoa, what is going on?"

I know how the baby got in there, but how does the baby get out?

I want to be there for my wife during labor. But I'm not sure how I'll handle it. I'm not that big on blood or pain, and I don't want to see her in pain.

I want to maximize my wife's comfort and make sure she and the baby are safe.

While women want their partners with them to share the birth, they often express concern about how their partner will handle labor. Three women in my prenatal yoga class shared their apprehensions:

I want my husband with me, but I'm not sure how he'll respond. I don't want to have to worry about how he's doing when I'm in labor.

In my first labor, my husband kept trying to help by telling me what to do. It really got in my way, and I remember thinking he didn't have a clue. This time I hope he gets it. I really want him there for me.

I want my husband's support. But if he gets tense, it will make it harder for me. I can't be dealing with my husband and labor too. He needs to know that.

By using the three-step, one-minute centering practice over and over again during labor, you remain centered and free your partner from having concerns about how you are doing. This is a great gift.

HOW TO COMMUNICATE WITH A LABORING WOMAN

When you communicate with your partner during labor, do it from the position of the integrated warrior, from an incorporated whole. Sherry shared: *When my husband talked to me in labor, I could tell exactly where he was coming from. When he was available and present, I could tell. Whatever he said, I could receive as support. But if he was coming from a mental place, no matter what he said, it sounded hollow. Even though he spoke supportive words, if he didn't feel it top-to-bottom in his own body, I didn't want to hear it.*

A woman in labor is not in a mental place. As a matter of fact, her rational mind shuts down. She is stripped to an essential and potent level of being. If you communicate with the mother from a mental place, it pulls her out of the intuitive space she needs to be in to manage labor. It also pulls you out of the centered space you need to be in to accurately observe and respond to her.

It is also wise not to touch or talk to the mother from an anxious or a distracted place. That burdens her, because she not only has her labor to contend with, but your anxious or distracted energy as well. If you touch or talk to your partner when you are anxious or distracted, she will immediately detect it, and it will distract, distress, and isolate her. Use your one-minute centering practice to establish your stability before communicating.

Touch is a powerful and immediate form of communication. Sometimes touch is exactly what your partner needs. When you touch her, do it from a calm, centered space. When you remain centered, you remain strong. This helps your partner find her center and strength, which in turn helps her to find her way through labor.

During labor the mother is in touch with, being guided by, and dealing with profound and powerful forces within. Do not underestimate the wisdom that directs the contractions. And do not underestimate the silent power of your mountain presence to assist your partner. However, do not take this as a prescription that you should be silent during labor. Sometimes your partner needs silence. But other times, she is buoyed by verbal encouragement. When you focus on her, you detect her changing needs. Whether you communicate with your partner through talk or touch, do it from your center—from the position of an integrated warrior.

HOLD THE SPACE

During labor your partner is pushed to her limit, or beyond. If you do something that distracts or annoys her, she may snap at you. When this happens, men frequently recoil. They think they are making it worse. They don't know how to *fix* it and they don't know what to *do*, so they withdraw.

Patricia described snapping at her husband and how his reaction affected her: *My husband kept talking to me, and his talking was not working for me. It was distracting and irritating. He kept telling me I was doing great. It was driving me crazy. I remember thinking, 'Don't tell me I'm doing great. I'm not doing great. I'm in labor. Don't you get it?' But it wasn't like I could talk and tell him the effect he was having on me. Finally, I snapped at him and told him to shut up. Then he backed off and pulled away. I thought, 'If you are going to play that trip, go. Get out of here. I have no space for being able to care take you right now.' What I needed from my husband was his presence, and that was it.*

Her husband Sam shared how he felt when she snapped at him, and then shared his important realization: *When my wife told me to shut up, I pulled back. I didn't know how to help her, and I felt like I was making it worse. So rather than worry about doing something wrong, I took myself out. Once I got that all she needed was for me to be there, it made so much more sense. It was easier for me not to have to think about what to say. It sounded so trivial anyway. And I had been preoccupied with what I should say next, instead of being focused on her.*

If your partner snaps at you, stop what you are doing. But don't doubt yourself. You are important to her, and she does not want you to withdraw or abandon her emotionally. She is doing the best she can to communicate. Experienced attendants get snapped at too, but they know not to take it personally. When a storm passes over a mountain, a mountain does not collapse; it holds the space. Use the one-minute centering technique to flow with it and recoup your equilibrium.

Guy recounted how staying centered helped his partner find the intuitive space she needed to be in to manage labor: *For me, labor was about learning how to stay centered. It kept me out of my own way, and it kept me out of her way. Without my telling her, she knew exactly where to go. She went into this intuitive laboring pregnant place without any help. That was a big lesson for me. It was interesting how she just knew where to go. When it did get really hard for her, I spoke, but it came from my being there instead of my telling her how to do it.*

This is an important understanding. Your centered presence holds the space and gives your partner the stable base she needs to find her own path.

ENDURANCE: A MOUNTAIN DOES NOT SPEND ITS STRENGTH

Men tend to demonstrate their strength in intense battle, whereas women tend to demonstrate their strength in endurance. Your partner needs endurance to get through labor. But so do you. Men have physical strength. However, labor tests their strength on all fronts: endurance, focus, fortitude, emotions, patience, and ability to deal with the unknown, as well as physical strength.

Jack was surprised by the level of endurance labor required from him: *I work in a gym and I'm in good shape, so I had no idea I would be the one who would barely make it through labor. I didn't expect to get hungry. I didn't expect to get sleep-deprived. I didn't expect my wife and I would get on each other's nerves. I'm a trainer, and I thought I'd be able to offer my wife some instruction and cheer her on. But it didn't work that way at all. The more I tried to help her, the more she shut down, until finally labor stalled. We both got discouraged and exhausted.*

If you try too hard to help your partner, chances are it will backfire. A mountain does not spend its strength; it contains the strength. It is potential, reserve. Let your partner draw upon your energy and strength as she needs it. It is not your job to figure out how to get your partner through labor, instruct her, or project your own agenda. It *is* your job to provide stability and refuge. In addition, when you use the one-minute centering practice to remain calm, it decreases your adrenaline levels. This helps to keep your partner's adrenaline levels lower, which contributes to making her contractions strong and productive.

Another example of how men spend their strength and exhaust themselves comes when they *throw* all their energy into massaging their partners' lower backs. Men can fall into the trap of feeling responsible for *fixing* it. They get trapped in the details, lose the larger perspective, and become unavailable in other meaningful ways. If a man's focus is on *fixing*, he is draining his energy in an attempt to fix something he cannot fix. It's labor. Men do not help their partners by exhausting themselves.

As an alternative to operating from effort and strength, use your weight to lean into your partner's lower back. Keep your breath flowing and your position as comfortable as possible. This allows you to provide counterpressure for her lower back, yet simultaneously remain accessible and responsive. To conserve your energy and maintain your stable presence, support her with your body weight, instead of your strength, whenever possible.

SUPPORT HER TO FIND HER OWN WAY

When you maintain your mountain and warrior presence, you more accurately perceive and respond to your partner's cues and support her to find her way. Jim described his method of being responsive: *Instead of talking to my wife and asking her if she wanted or needed anything, I observed her and responded to her cues and requests. I supported her to find her own way, but we worked together as a team. There were times when it got really intense. That meant I had to be responsive in the moment. If I saw something that would help my wife get through her contraction, I did it. I didn't talk to her about it. But I observed her reaction to make sure what I was doing was what she needed.*

To manage labor, a woman needs to stay seated in the instinctive, intuitive aspect of her being. A woman who manages labor well goes into a trance state, and you do not want to draw her out of it. Having to use her rational mind to respond to questions or instructions forces her out of the intuitive space she needs to be in and makes labor more difficult.

Henry shared how using the one-minute centering practice over and over again during labor helped him to focus on his partner: *I could feel myself getting wrapped up in, 'Am I doing this right?' I had to keep dropping that and return to the centering practice so I could focus on her and not be so anxious about whether I was doing it right.*

When you respond from your center, you help her find her center. This opens up a greater possibility for her to dive deep to uncover whatever she needs to manage labor. Jennifer shared her experience with diving deep: *As soon as I dove in, everything changed. I went deep, deep into this timeless space between worlds, and I was with my baby. My baby communicated to me that pain is what grounds you here, and that I shouldn't be afraid of it. She let me know clearly: no matter what happens, it's okay. I experienced this profound acceptance, completely void of any drama or pain, and it was expansive.*

Your centered companionship is instrumental in supporting your partner so she can draw what she needs from her internal resources to manage labor and have the most rewarding experience possible.

LOSING IT AND FINDING THE WAY

Mountain and warrior energy give your partner the support and protection needed to navigate labor without having other concerns. It gives her the freedom to be honest. To lose her confidence. To get a little crazy, if she needs to—sometimes we have to get crazy so we don't go crazy. And then come back.

If your partner cannot fall apart in the heat, enormity, and depth of labor, where can she fall apart? I know it sounds strange, but losing it, falling, getting lost in the midst of the ocean of labor can be exactly what your partner needs to uncover her inner compass and find her path through the remainder. Getting lost is how we discover our individual paths.

If your partner loses it in labor, she needs you (more than ever) to be the mountain that stands through the storm without collapse. Holding the space during intense times is easier said than done. It is a giant offering on your part. In later chapters, you will get more tools to assist your partner through the *I don't know if I can do this* times.

DIVE INTO THE BREATH

Sometimes the situation gets so heated you cannot be stable like the mountain and agile like the warrior, and you lose it. Ken shared: *At one point, my wife shut down from exhaustion and pain. It was hard to see her in such discomfort. I didn't know how to give her what she needed, and I felt frantic.* If you get frantic, collect yourself before acting. Avoid the urge to assist your partner from a place of *needing to do something* to relieve your own anxieties.

Tom shared: *In the middle of labor, my wife was in so much pain that I had never seen her like that. No one had told me it could get that bad. I was desperate to help her. But I was so beside myself that instead of helping, I made it worse.* If you become desperate, you are a disturbance to yourself and your partner. Now she not only has her labor to contend with, but she has you to contend with as well. Things can quickly spiral downward from this point; you can both get caught in it.

It is easier for your partner to cope if you are vulnerable and honest than it is if you try to *do something* or *hold it together* from a frantic, desperate, or rigid space. Vulnerability and honesty are huge factors in strength. Give yourself the freedom to fall.

Imposing impossible standards on yourself when you cannot do it is like following a useless script. If you find yourself derailed in the midst of labor, know you can be tested and fail. And still succeed. Sages are sages because they have failed more than the rest of us and have continued. Failure is part of success. (As a matter of fact, failure may be the only true path to success.)

If you find yourself reacting rigidly to a particularly challenging part of labor, like a deer frozen in headlights, you know you are operating from your unconsciously motivated habitual format. Instead of trying to help, dive into your breathing. It's a shorter version of the three-step, one-minute centering practice. Let go of everything and connect to the breath. Think of the phrase attributed to Lao Tse, a founder of Taoism: *Be still like a mountain and flow like a great river.* Be still, drop your armor, and focus on your breath until it is fluid and rhythmic.

In a panic situation, once your breath is flowing, it regulates your nervous system and stabilizes you. Then you can respond from a place of stability, instead of reacting from a place of needing to relieve your anxieties. If you establish your breath and still do not know how to help, know that less is more. Sometimes the most valuable contribution you can make in the moment is simply to dive into your breath and be there. Surprisingly, how you breathe not only has a profound influence on you, but on those around you. Few things in life are as comforting or reassuring as the sound and movement of smooth, rhythmic breath.

CHAPTER 4
BREATH: THE KEY TO REDUCING PAIN

BREATH: KEEP IT FLOWING

Other than your mountain and warrior presence, your most important contribution to labor is helping your partner keep her breath flowing. Tension and anxiety increase the minute breath becomes shallow or restricted, and decrease the minute breath becomes smooth and flowing. Breath is the most powerful tool you can use to keep you both centered. It is also the most powerful tool your partner can use to decrease pain.

The first action you take in any situation is a breath. The breath affects the lungs, immediately cueing the nervous system. The nervous system responds by sending messages, which impact the mind-body system. Messages sent from the nervous system affect us physically, emotionally, and mentally. If we alter how we breathe, we alter the constellation of messages and reactions in our entire system.

A focus on the breath keeps you both grounded in the moment, and gives each of you the ability to work with one wave of labor at a time. You cannot breathe in the past or in the future. By focusing on the breath, you help your partner stay focused in the now. Most women can deal with one breath, one wave of labor at a time. When a woman cannot release tension from one wave, she carries it into the next wave. As tension accumulates from one wave to the next, labor becomes overwhelming. Then the mother either accelerates or shuts down the breath in an effort to cope.

Rapid, shallow breathing, hyperventilating, or temporarily holding the breath seems to help the mother cope in the moment. But the result is escalating pain, which creates a downward spiral. Simple intervention with her breath prevents it from continuing. Rhythmic, flowing breath helps the mother release tension between the waves, as well as *during* the waves, which reduces pain.

When breath is haphazard, rapid, shallow, or exhibits long pauses, it cues the nervous system to release fright, flight, or fight responses. Then tension, anxiety, and pain levels soar. Getting through labor with recurrent fright, flight, or fight cues is like scaling a cliff that goes straight up with no rope to hold onto. The minute you assist your partner to focus on breath, it is like giving her a rope so she can continue her climb. (*See* Chapter 10 for Breath Intervention Skills.)

Julie shared how important it was to have her partner assist her with breath: *I couldn't have made it through labor without drugs if my husband hadn't been there to keep me focused on the breath. It helped me to anchor whenever I panicked.*

Effective breathing is critical for your partner, but how you breathe can make a big difference in the effectiveness of your contribution. Your stable presence is anchored in your own fluid breathing. Alexander shared how breath was a key element during his labor vigil: *Labor was like this giant observance of the breath—both my breath and my wife's. The breath kept us connected. By keeping tabs on my breath, I kept connected to myself and by keeping tabs on her breath, I kept connected to her and how she was doing. And it really is true; there are few things as stabilizing or reassuring as flowing breath.*

Simply diving into your breath has a profound influence on you both. Breath literally has the power to revolutionize your experience.

THE GREAT AND SIMPLE TEACHING OF BREATH

Breath is the link between body and mind. You can relax a tense body or focus an agitated or distracted mind when you attend the breath and allow it to be:

- Diaphragmatic
- Flowing without exaggerated breaks
- Smooth and fluid, without jerks or restrictions
- Quiet, refined, without noises (This does not mean your partner should not combine the exhalation with groaning during her waves—more on that later.)

Do not be deceived by the simplicity of this practice. The simplest practices are the most powerful and profound. Fluid, rhythmic, diaphragmatic breathing is so effective that within forty seconds, a biofeedback machine records the body's physiological alteration. I witnessed this when I went through a series of biofeedback sessions as part of a holistic therapy program. Tension levels measurably decrease, and body temperature measurably increases, indicating enhanced levels of relaxation. This is called the *relaxation response.*

Breath is intimately connected to the nervous system, which immediately affects your entire psychophysiological system. Breath has the power to turn an unnerving situation around in less than a minute. Engaging the relaxation response by rhythmic, smooth breathing is the most powerful tool you and your partner can use during labor.

When breath is diaphragmatic and flows smoothly, without exaggerated breaks or restrictions, it is physiologically not possible to be in a state of agitation. This is not a belief system. It is a practice. I ask my clients not to simply believe this, but to *use* it to discover whether or not it is true. (*See* Chapter 14 for Simple Breath Practices.)

BREATH AND ALIGNMENT

The quality of breath is intimately connected to alignment. Misalignment inhibits effective breathing, creates unnecessary tension, detrimentally affects body organs, and requires the body to use additional energy to support its weight and position. If your partner's breath is constricted because of collapsed alignment, she not only has to cope with the powerful force of labor, but also with the emotional impact of the nervous system firing fight, flight, or fright cues. One way you help ease this impossible cycle is by attending your partner's alignment.

Comfortable alignment supports the mother to breathe more proficiently, reduces a measure of discomfort, and conserves energy. By keeping the mother as aligned, supported, and comfortable as is practical, you increase her ability to breathe and relax.

THE MECHANICS OF ALIGNMENT

The body has three basic weights: pelvis, chest, and head. Observe the mother's alignment from time to time and help keep these three body weights as aligned, supported, and comfortable as is practical. Think in terms of observing and supporting her whole body, from the crown of her head to the tips of her toes. The position of the spine is pivotal because it reflects alignment of pelvis, chest, and head. She will need periodic support of her head, lower back, and legs. Use pillows or rolled towels for additional support when needed. (See Chapters 14–16 for more detailed information on how to support your partner's alignment during labor.)

However, don't get trapped in the details of alignment and lose the larger perspective. Too much attention to detail will annoy and distract your partner. Supported comfort is the main idea.

KEEP HER BODY WARM

Another easy way you contribute to your partner's alignment and breath flow is to keep her warm. A chilly body cannot relax. If the mother gets chilly, her muscles contract, which causes misalignment, unnecessary tension, restricted breath flow, and increased pain. When your partner is in deep labor, she may not realize on the rational level that she is cold. It is your job to ensure she is not.

Warmth conveys nurture and safety. If your partner gets chilly, she releases adrenaline, which inhibits oxytocin, the hormone that sustains labor. The caring act of keeping your partner warm supports alignment, breath flow, and encourages labor to progress with more ease. Cover her with an extra blanket, and offer hot packs.

There may be times when your partner feels hot. Offer an ice pack to place on her forehead or neck. Keeping the mother's body temperature comfortable is one way to support her.

DETAILS ON BREATH

A BRIEF OVERVIEW ON THE ANATOMY OF BREATH

Lungs cannot move without muscle action. The diaphragm is designed to be the main breathing muscle. It is shaped like a large dome (think upside-down bowl) that separates the chest cavity from the abdominal cavity. The diaphragm works in conjunction with the intercostal chest muscles that expand and contract the lower ribs during diaphragmatic breathing. Optimally, the diaphragm moves downward with the inhalation and upward with the exhalation. Like a pump, it distributes energy through the body, and its movement massages and tones the organs. A breath pattern that restricts or reverses fluid movement of the diaphragm increases tension in the entire system.

CHEST VERSUS DIAPHRAGMATIC BREATHING

If the primary movement of breath is in the upper chest, breath is shallower and faster, which creates anxiety and tension, and requires more muscle action and energy. Chest breathing restricts movement of the diaphragm, limiting its ability to work as a pump. Because of the inefficient distribution of energy throughout the body, it creates a host of other problems. Diaphragmatic breathing uses less energy, is the most efficient and effective way for the body to habitually breathe, is calming, benefits the entire mind-body system, and is often referred to as the *anti-anxiety breath*.

The author of *Radical Healing : Integrating the World's Great Therapeutic Traditions to Create a New Transformative Medicine*, Rudolph Ballantine, MD, who was my teacher and homeopathic physician, explained the opposing effect diaphragmatic versus chest breathing has on the nervous system: *Moving the most breath with the least effort, diaphragmatic breathing involves gentle expansion at the midriff that is quieting and calming. How it affects emotions might be understood physiologically if we look at the impact of breath on the autonomic nervous system, which gears you up (sympathetic) or down (parasympathetic). For example, chest breathing creates sympathetic arousal: By design, the chest is drawn strongly into action only when unusually large amounts of oxygen are needed—during exertion for example, or in emergencies. Breathing primarily with the chest tends to set off a chain reaction of physiological events that say: 'Prepare yourself; something is about to happen!'*[1]

BELLY BREATHING

Many people think belly, or abdominal, breathing is deep breathing. However, the body breathes more deeply and efficiently when the predominant rise and fall is located in the diaphragm region, immediately above the navel, rather than in the abdominal region. During belly breathing, the focus is on making the belly inflate. If you try belly breathing, you discover it takes more energy and muscle action to breathe abdominally than it does diaphragmatically.

When your partner is in labor, the abdomen is the location of major uterine contraction. While there is gentle movement in the belly during diaphragmatic breathing, inflating the belly with the breath is exhausting. Your partner will find it more soothing during labor if she focuses on the movement of her breath immediately above the navel in the diaphragm region.

THE NUMBERS

A healthy adult is capable of surviving weeks without food and days without water, but only minutes without oxygen. Extensive information is available on the quality and quantity of nutrition and fluids required to maintain health, but little information is widely available on the quality of breath and its direct affect on health. Oxygen is the critical underlying factor that sustains life, and the nourishment of respiration occurs on the cellular level. Breath is the prime mover. No breath, no life.

CHAPTER 4

Let's consider how many times a day a body breathes. While there are no conclusive studies, most people breathe 14 to 24 times per minute. Some shallow breathers average 32 times per minute or more; some diaphragmatic breathers average 10 times per minute or less.

Suppose a man has an average rate of 17 breaths per minute. He breathes 1,020 times per hour, 24,480 times a day. The numbers speak for themselves. Breath is a continual action, a constant movement. Now suppose he becomes a more conscious, diaphragmatic breather. His habitual breath pattern drops to 13 breaths per minute, 780 times per hour, 18,720 times a day. He now breathes 240 fewer times per hour. Multiply that by days, weeks, months, and years, and you see of the reduction of work the body must do to keep itself inspired with breath's nourishment.

Breath is also the main pathway the body uses for cleansing. Much of the body's wastes are exhaled with the breath. The more efficiently you breathe, the more your body is able to nourish and cleanse, to heal and maintain health.

BREATH, HEART, AND HEALTH

Breath and heart are so closely connected that we often refer to the *cardiorespiratory* system. The lower surface of the heart rests directly on the diaphragm. Thus the rhythm and movement of the diaphragm directly affects the heart. The heart is the main generator of electrical energy in the body.

Electrocardiograms measure and record the pattern of electrical energy generated by the heart. The pattern of cardiographic traces is directly connected to the pattern of the breath. A haphazard, unconscious, choppy breath pattern increases unease. It also creates choppy and haphazard electrical impulses generated by the heart.[2] A rhythmic, smooth, diaphragmatic breath increases ease. It also creates smoother, more rhythmic electrical impulses generated by the heart.[3] Over the course of a lifetime, the direct impact of breath pattern on the pattern of electrical energy generated by the heart is enormous, and may affect heart as well as overall health.

Thoughts and emotions are intimately connected to breath. Anger, resentment, grief, fear, joy, love, and gratitude affect the quality of breath; these emotions also affect the quality of electrical impulses generated by the heart. Because breath is intimately connected to your physical, as well as your emotional and mental health, how you breathe influences your overall health. Justin O'Brien, PhD, author of *The Wellness Tree : The Dynamic Six-Step Program for Creating Optimal Wellness,* and one of my teachers, comments: *Diaphragmatic breathing disrupts chronic stress patterns, enabling the body's innate healing force to mobilize its energy.*[4]

BREATH CAN BE EITHER CONSCIOUS OR UNCONSCIOUS

Our bodies continue breathing whether we pay attention or not. Breath can be either participatory and conscious or involuntary and unconscious. Unlike the heartbeat, breath is an easy instrument to bring into conscious awareness. Donna Farhi, a yoga teacher I studied with, and author of *The Breathing Book,* said: *At one end of the breath is the unconscious, involuntary breath; at the other end is breathing that is controlled and regulated by the will.... Between these two extremes lies the 'essential' breath, a conscious flow that arises out of the depth of our being and dissolves effortlessly back into our core.*[5]

Conscious use of breath is a tool we can use to bring our system back into balance. It is a tool we can use to dispel anxiety and clouded thinking. Because breath is literally connected to every action, becoming a more effective breather has exponential results. It affects everything—from digestion to tension, to how you handle challenges, and more. The simplest changes are the most profound. If you become a more conscious, diaphragmatic breather, you will you reap the rewards, and so will everyone around you.

BREATH IS LIFE

Deep inside, you know breath is life. Inhalation is the first independent action your baby takes. That first breath is the demarcation line; it is the thread that draws us into life and the vital element that protects and ensures our crossing. From this perspective, breath is life. Life begins with the first inspiration and ends with the last expiration. While we have life, breath is our constant companion. It accompanies us wherever we go, whatever we do. It does not abandon us.

If we have a haphazard, erratic, unconscious, shallow chest-breath pattern, we have a constant companion that is continually disturbing us. If we have a smooth, conscious, flowing diaphragmatic breath pattern, we have a constant companion that is continually supporting us. Breath has the compassion and the wisdom to support and assist us. Having a good practice and developing an ongoing relationship with breath is of great value.

BABY'S BREATH
All babies use the diaphragm to breathe. Babies come into the world the least developed of all mammals. Because the nervous system is not sufficiently developed at birth for them to use the intercostal muscles of the chest, babies cannot chest breathe.[6] After your baby is born, you may note his respiration rate is more rapid than yours— around forty to fifty times per minute.

SUMMARY ON THE POWER OF BREATH
- Breath is the link between body and mind.
- The body is optimally designed to breathe diaphragmatically.
- You can calm and relax a tense body using the breath.
- You can focus an agitated, dissipated, or distracted mind using the breath.
- Diaphragmatic breathing reduces anxiety, tension, and pain. It positively affects health and emotions, and may reduce high blood pressure, heart attack risk, and more.
- Smooth, diaphragmatic breath measurably alters the body's physiology in less than a minute. Tension decreases and body temperature rises, indicating a relaxation response.
- Breath is both a voluntary and an involuntary function. You continue to breathe whether you pay attention or not. But breath is easily brought into conscious awareness. Through conscious use of the breath, you have the power to influence your entire system.
- Your breath is your constant companion. It can be a constant source of either subliminal disturbance or support. Habitual, shallow, chest breathing generates underlying disturbance. Habitual, synchronized, diaphragmatic breathing generates underlying support.
- The breath and the nervous system are intimately connected. Shallow, erratic, chest breathing cues fight, flight, or fright responses. Smooth, flowing diaphragmatic breathing calms the nervous system and increases well-being.

- When breath is diaphragmatic and flows rhythmically without restrictions or breaks, it is physiologically not possible to be in a state of agitation.
- Your individual breath pattern influences your nervous system, your health, your personality, your tension levels, your thoughts, and your psychophysiology.
- The simple but profound truth is, when you alter your breath, you alter your life.

OPPOSITE EXPERIENCES:
THE DIFFERENCE PRACTICE MAKES

How you and your partner use breath during labor dramatically influences how it unfolds and can alter the outcome of the birth. Here are two birth stories from the same couple, Joan and Gerald, that demonstrate the difference breath, practice, and preparation can make:

We attended classes, but we learned facts instead of the how. When my wife went into labor, we knew we needed to breathe and focus. But we didn't know how to do it, and we both got anxious. Just when I thought it couldn't get worse, my wife started to hyperventilate. I had no idea what to do or how to help. That's when the nurse came in and asked if she was ready for an epidural. It seemed like the only way out, so we took it. After the epidural, we got some relief for a while. But when it was time to push, she had trouble pushing, and they got the forceps out. I was stunned as I watched those things go inside my wife's body. They tried to pull the baby out, but he wouldn't come. Then there was this crisis flurry of activity, and they whisked her off for emergency surgery. No one even spoke to me. I was left standing outside alone. But when I saw the baby, I was amazed by how perfect he was.

The following story is from the same couple, after I helped them prepare for their second birth:

My wife exercised and practiced breathing and relaxation during pregnancy in her prenatal yoga class. We practiced labor in our couples' class, and I practiced some breathing and relaxation too. When my wife went into labor, I got a little anxious and so did she. But we were able to calm ourselves down by using our breath and other skills. I was surprised they actually worked. I felt good about how we worked to-gether. Pushing went pretty fast for her. Then the baby just slipped out. I can't describe how great it was. I was relieved everything had gone so well. It was a high that lasted for weeks.

Through preparation and practice, most couples can avoid scenarios like Gerald's first birth experience or like the first experience that Robert, another of my clients, described:

When my wife's labor got painful, I panicked. She was the one holding my hand, supporting me, and telling me it would be all right. (Isn't it supposed to work the other way?) I was worse than useless. I remember thinking men should not be involved in birth. What happened next, I don't even want to tell you. The nurse said, 'Come take a look. The baby is crowning.' I took one look, and heard my wife saying, 'Honey, focus. Breathe.' Then I passed out. When I came to, there was blood everywhere. They put me on a gurney and rolled me away. By the time they cleaned and stitched me up and I got back to the room, the whole thing was over. I wish I could have been there for her.

Robert also recounted his second birth experience:

When my wife got pregnant a second time, I didn't want to attend the birth, but she insisted I try it again. This time we took a couples' class where we practiced breathing, relaxation, and skills for labor. We asked the teacher to come to our birth. Learning how to breathe made a huge difference. I wouldn't have believed that. But what also made a difference was having the birth assistant with us. She knew what was going on, and helped us stay grounded, calm, and connected. When my baby was born, I was so thankful I was there and didn't miss it. After the birth, my wife and I did so much better. We felt like we could work together as a team after all.

These examples illustrate the difference breath practices make. By using diaphragmatic breathing, you remain more relaxed. The more relaxed you remain, the more it helps your partner relax. The more she relaxes, the less pain she experiences.

Practice can result in a peak experience, much like Richard had: *Being there to greet my son at the precise moment he was born was an indescribable and extraordinary privilege. I was swept into this high, but I was really clear. It was like opening a door and meeting my real self and my son at the same time.*

Integrating your body, breath, and mind by using the one-minute centering practice unleashes the capacity you have within. It gives you the focus you need to marshal your energy and achieve your potential. But the greatest gift of practice is that it introduces you to the truth of your own being.

CHAPTER 5
RELAXATION AND THE TRUTH WITHIN

RESISTANCE AND RELAXATION

It is a natural human tendency to resist force with force. However, during labor, this natural tendency is counterproductive. The more a mother resists labor, the more pain escalates. Forced effort reduces effectiveness, whereas a relaxed, willing-to-receive openness produces better results.

Resistance, effort, determination, and strength can be deceptive. On occasion, the determination and strength of our will helps us persevere through a trying or relentless situation so we don't retreat or abandon our purpose. At other times, the determination and effort of our individual will makes the situation less yielding and more hazardous, lessening our chances of success.

If you think of how the ocean surf crashes with roaring force into a rock wall that lines the shore, but how that same surf washes onto a sandy shoreline in rhythmic waves, you have a picture of how resisting the natural flow makes labor more difficult.

You can both use this image in labor. Go to the beach. Lie low. Give way. Your partner lets the waves of labor wash over and through her without resistance. A similar image is the warrior concept of rolling with the punches. When you are struck by a blow, yielding saves you from injury.

SYNTHESIS: CONTRACTION AND EXPANSION

We live in a world of duality, of opposites. Movement, growth, and opening occur because of opposition, but from another perspective, movement, growth, and opening occur because of harmony. This is a paradox. When you bend your finger, one set of muscles contracts, but another set of equal and opposing muscles expands. In labor, the large and powerful uterine muscle contracts, which expands and opens the cervix. From one perspective, it is opposition, contraction; from another perspective, it is harmony, expansion. It's an equal and opposing synthesis, a dance.

Because the purpose of contraction in labor is to expand and open the cervix, a wave of labor is simultaneously a contraction and an expansion. The contraction is good and necessary. The expansion is good and necessary. Both are purposeful and needed components. Birth is the synthesis of contraction and expansion.

BENEFICIAL ASPECTS OF CONTRACTION

Contraction concentrates and magnifies power. It also armors and protects. When your partner is in labor, powerful forces convene to contract the uterus. This contracted power has authority and wisdom. The contraction is the one essential component that opens the cervix and moves the baby through the birth canal to be born. No contraction, no expansion. No movement, no birth.

The contraction is potent, and it will do its work with or without assistance. Your partner does not want to gather her energy to work against this convening, wise force. That approach exhausts her and makes the labor longer and more painful. This is why your assistance to help your partner focus, breathe, and relax *during* the contraction, as well as between contractions, is so important to her. (*See* Chapters 10 and 11 for strategies to help her focus, breathe, and relax.)

LABOR IS EXPANSION

The truth of labor is expansion. Its purpose is to open (expand) the cervix wide enough for the baby to pass through. Labor's goal is to get the cervix softened, thinned, and opened enough for your partner to push your baby into the world. If you connect to labor as contraction, it will not help your partner expand and open. Think of labor as expansion, opening.

RUNNING AND THE EYE OF THE HURRICANE

When I was in India, walking alone through the small remaining portion of jungle outside the city of Rishikesh, I saw an elephant in the wild. My first reaction, without thinking, was to turn and run away as fast as I could. Your partner's body may respond to labor by wanting to run away. However, she cannot escape labor; the only way out is through.

Think of the centrifugal force in a hurricane. As you move away from the eye of a hurricane, the force gets stronger. If your partner attempts to run, she encounters a more powerful force. The way to stop running and get out of the centrifugal force is to dive into the center, into the eye of the storm. If you help her dive into her breathing, you give her a way back in—and out of the centrifugal force.

THE TRUTH WITHIN AND SOFT GAZING

Discovering you both are already equipped with innate wisdom and resources to guide you gives you more confidence to trust in the wise process of labor. The yellow circle experiment, described below, uses soft gazing to help you experience your access to knowledge within. To verify you have access to knowledge you didn't know you knew, consider this question: What is the complement of the color yellow?

The truth is everyone knows the complement of yellow, but not everyone knows they know. Use soft gazing and relaxation to discover the complement of yellow. In my birthing class, I pass out white sheets of cardboard with a yellow circle printed on them. In the center of the circle is a black dot. If you choose, make one on your computer and print it out.

To begin, experiment with hard gazing. Stare intently at the black dot in the center of the yellow circle. Focus hard. Concentrate exactly on the point. Note the increased tension in the forehead and eyes. The more the eyes tense, the more the body tenses, and the more restricted breath becomes. If you focus hard, you use effort, but it is unlikely you will see the radiating complementary color flashing off the edges of the yellow circle.

A hard gaze takes more effort, increases tension, drains energy, and limits your ability to receive internal guidance and respond to your partner's cues. It also restricts your view, which decreases your ability to head off unnecessary disruption for your partner. A mountain does not strain to view the horizon.

Next, experiment with soft gazing. Sit comfortably with soft eyes and a wide-open gaze. Softly focus on the yellow circle, while your gaze simultaneously takes in the dot, the circle, and the expanded view beyond the circle. Relax. Do not work or strain. The eye is the window to the body. When the eye relaxes, the whole body relaxes and the breath naturally begins to flow.

After a few moments of soft gazing, you effortlessly see the complementary color (iridescent violet) radiating off the edges of the yellow circle. For those clients who didn't know the complement of yellow, discovering they have access to knowledge they didn't know they knew is an eye-opener. For those who previously knew, discovering they have a direct path to knowledge without having to be instructed is also an eye-opener.

SOFT GAZE APPROACH

Soft gazing helps to keep you relaxed during your labor vigil. It allows you to be aware of your partner with less effort, so you can more accurately perceive and respond to her cues. It also broadens your view so you can protect the space and provide a buffer.

Both of you can use this approach to labor: soft gaze (although your partner may prefer to softly close her eyes to focus within), fluid breath, and relaxed and receptive body. These are the same qualities you use when you see violet radiating off the edges of the yellow circle. Use soft gazing to avoid the impossible task of trying to be in control.

RELAXATION DECREASES RESISTANCE: CORNSTARCH PLAY

Experiencing kinesthetically that relaxation decreases resistance helps you both understand relaxation's value. In some instances, what you cannot accomplish with effort, you can easily accomplish with relaxation. The cornstarch experiment, described below, helps you learn on a kinesthetic level the truth that relaxation decreases resistance.

To do this experiment, pour a one-pound box of cornstarch into a large bowl. Slowly add a small amount of water, and stir the mixture with a spoon until it is the consistency of smooth, thick paste. If the consistency is too thin, this experiment will not work. If you added too much water, let the cornstarch sit until the water rises to the surface. Then you can pour off the excess water, and stir to a thick paste.

Tighten your fingers together and make your hand rigid. Deliver quick, forceful jabs to the surface of the cornstarch mixture. No matter how much force you use, the cornstarch resists forceful attempts to penetrate it. Next, relax and rest the weight of your hand on the surface of the cornstarch. Your hand sinks right into it without effort—it offers no resistance.

Couples are surprised to discover that what they could not accomplish with effort and strength, they can easily accomplish with relaxation and effortlessness. Jennifer, one of my clients who tried the cornstarch demonstration in class, commented after her birth:

The cornstarch image stayed with me all through labor. It helped me get out of my own way so I could let go and let it happen.

MUSCLE TISSUE ACTS LIKE CORNSTARCH

Muscle tissue acts surprisingly like cornstarch. If you force a muscle to stretch, the muscle responds by resisting and contracting. However, if you move to the edge of a comfortable stretch, then stop, breathe, draw back slightly, and relax, the muscle does not fire receptors that cause it to contract. You can then release into a deeper stretch with less effort and achieve a fuller range of motion without the damage, pain, or resistance of forcing a muscle.

The uterus is a powerful muscle. The more the mother resists labor, the more pain she experiences, and the more unyielding the cervix may become. Conversely, the more she relaxes, the less pain she experiences, and the more yielding the cervix may become. The more relaxed you remain, the more it encourages your partner to relax. Use cornstarch play to kinesthetically learn relaxation decreases resistance.

CHAPTER 6
THE TRANSCENDENT POWER OF BIRTH

CONCEPTION

As a couple, some of you made a decision to have a baby. However, making a decision to have a baby and acting on that decision doesn't ensure a conception. Some of you were shocked to find out your partner was pregnant. Deciding not to have a baby, at least not now, doesn't ensure your partner won't conceive. Some of you know exactly when it happened, and some of you are still wondering.

What you *want* or *choose* or *decide* is not entirely what pregnancy is about. Something deeper is going on. The rational mind is crucial, but you are more than a decision-making being. Neither of you use the rational mind to oversee the intricate development of your baby. You don't decide when or how to develop the fingers or whether the baby has a dimple. It is not about you and your partner and what the two of you want.

In pregnancy, birthing, and fathering, you are given a corporal opportunity to participate with the mystery that is in us and among us. One form of the mystery is the pregnant body. How is it that two people join together in sexual union and become one in conception? And how is it that one body becomes two (or more) in pregnancy? Jared said it like this: *It was kind of mind-blowing for me when I found out my wife was pregnant. I mean, how is it that two people become three?*

Conception is the contact point where separate, yet connected realms unite. The absolute and the manifest become one at conception. At the moment of conception, potential being explodes into action and is suddenly corporal and growing. What was not, transforms into the state of becoming. The fetus, this evolving microcosmic universe, forms with a little assistance from us. But mostly, we stand in awe of it. We are humbled by it.

We are all birthed through a mother body. The physical body is extraordinarily valuable. No body, no birth. Your partner's pregnant body is your baby's first Mother Earth. Care for the mother.

CHAPTER 6

KAIROS TIME

Birth is an expected, but unscheduled phenomenon. It occurs in what the ancient Greeks called *kairos time*. Kairos time is event time, time when Providence and earth collide, and life is forever changed. You cannot schedule or mark on your calendar the time labor will begin because it does not begin in linear time you plan or control; it is an event that happens in its own time. In ripened time. In strategic, life-altering time.

You get drawn out of chronos time and get catapulted into kairos time, where you have a rare opportunity to participate directly with the mystery. Encountering the mystery alters life and how you view and live it. On the day your child is born, you are born as father. The old order comes crashing down, and, simultaneously, the new order is initiated.

Ben said it like this: *We didn't need to take the baby home for the experience to change my life. Just seeing my son for the first time was an instantaneous altering of pretty much everything. The amazing thing is how overwhelmed I was, and how I felt this desire to protect him.*

Anthony said: *Seeing my baby for the first time was kind of like seeing the moment when you know your life is going to change forever. You know that going into it. I mean, it's obvious things are changing during the pregnancy. But when the precise moment happens, it takes you by surprise—the magnitude of it—meeting this person for the first time, while this person is entering the world.*

When you become a father, who you know yourself to be is permanently changed. You are initiated into the lineage of fathers as ancient as the beginning of man, and you share a link to all fathers in all times who have experienced love for their children. You are linked to the past, but you also hold an influential position that affects future generations. You are directly connected to and invested in the welfare of the next generation.

The day your child is born is a watershed, a permanent marker that rocks you to the core. Joel remembered: *To me, birth was like a grand initiation. It was like waking up to a whole new aspect of life I had never seen before and I didn't know existed.*

Bill shared: *Labor is like a long tunnel. When you enter the tunnel, you keep moving through, but it's dark and you can't see where you're going. Everything, except what is happening in that moment, goes away. Once we got to the other side, there were three of us instead of two.*

Bernard said: *Birth was a little like a near-death experience. I have actually had a near-death experience. And when I came back into my body, everything had shifted. What I thought was important before was no longer so important. And what I didn't know before, I knew. Plus, I was really thankful. Birth is like that experience.*

The power of a direct encounter with truth occurring in a kairos event like birth dismantles and reincorporates life as you know it. Birth is one of the few times when you cannot trade the truth for the counterfeit. It's an arrow that hits its mark. It transforms you instantly from the inside out.

TRIED BY FIRE: THE TRANSFORMATION

Birthing is so global that it is beyond what either of you anticipates. Frank shared: *Our birth plan, which my wife had put so much time into, became nonexistent once real labor hit. I remember thinking, 'As if we could plan our way through this.' No way could I have imagined the gripping power my wife was held in.*

Cara, his wife, shared: *When labor is in your body, it dwarfs any assumptions you may have had. I was shaken to the bone and stripped to the core. I traveled through labor with whatever grit and grace I could summon from the depths within me.*

Do not be deceived. Not only the women are tried by fire; so are the men. Below, Eric, Max, and Lawrence each comment on being tested during labor:

My wife pressed to her limit and beyond. And so was I. Labor was all about survival—my survival and hers and, of course, the baby's. But during labor, the birth seemed external, like it wasn't even a part of what was going on. I mean birth is such a short moment in time. And when it happens, everyone is focused on it. But the experience of labor was so big that I almost forgot it was about birth. It was all about both of us surviving the contraction she was having right in that minute.

I barely supported myself through labor. You'd expect a grown man to know there would be blood and body secretions, but it was more graphic, gritty, and even more violent than I thought it would be. But no matter what, I wouldn't have missed the birth. I held my baby right after she was born and that was all it took. I fell madly in love with her. She was so beautiful and so perfect, and my wife and I were so thankful we both cried.

I was amazed by how tremendously demanding labor was for me, because when you think about it, labor was not about me at all. I mean, it wasn't happening to me. It wasn't in my body. So for me, it meant not taking anything personally. It meant getting out of my own way and getting out of her way. And it meant focusing entirely on something that at the moment wasn't about me.

Even though labor is not going on in your body, you are still going through a form of labor—a major transition. Because you are intimately involved with your partner and baby, what happens to them, in effect, happens to you. Deep inside, men know this. Tom expressed it like this: *Safety is primary. I have a lot to do. It's hard to comprehend it.*

Of course your baby is the greatest gift of labor. But another great gift is you are pressed to your max or beyond, and you succeed. It expands who you know yourself to be. Jonah put it this way: *Labor is all about finding your threshold and learning you can go beyond it. It was certainly true for my wife, but it was also true for me.*

If your partner feels, for whatever reason, that labor did not unfold as she had hoped, she needs your assurance. No woman should be judged or judge herself for doing whatever she has to do to bring her baby forth into this world. And no man should be judged or judge himself for how he attends his partner or how he responds to birth. You are dealing with life on the edge. You do not know what will happen in it, and you are not in control. Together, you are participants in the mystery, and you do the best you can. The bottom line is your hope for a healthy baby and a healthy mom.

No matter how you do it, the power of birth expands your life. Jason said: *I was left with the gnawing sense there was a greater truth to be told. Not only did I have more regard and respect for my wife and women in general, but I had a greater regard and respect for my capacity and life itself. I had passed through the cavern of labor with my wife and life would never be the same. Our life was no longer just our own.*

On some levels, it doesn't matter how you both get through labor. There is no prescription. No script. No right way. Its commanding power does not depend exclusively on you or your partner to *do* it. No matter how you get through, it alters and expands you.

Your partner can go through labor immersed, submerged, and focused. Or she can go through screaming, whining, cussing, or fighting all the way. She can go through with or without drugs, conscious or not. Whether the birth is vaginal or cesarean; whether you are powerfully present, totally absent, or anywhere in between; birth deposits its power into your lives. The transformation is enduring. You can never go back.

COMMITMENT AND LOVE

In the first moments or days of your baby's life, you cross a barrier, and maybe for the first time, you discover your capacity to unconditionally commit yourself to another. You effortlessly and instinctively make an abiding commitment to your baby's welfare. Commitment is love in action. You do not commit because you have read about it or because someone said you should. You do not love your baby because of a logical argument or an idealistic concept. The love is not a debatable issue.

You know that you love your baby because you encounter it in the backbone of who you are. It is stamped in your fiber. You are clear. There is no doubt in it. Mitch shared his experience:

I didn't expect to immediately fall in love with my daughter and feel so protective of her the minute she was born. They used a syringe to get the mucus out, and they wouldn't stop using it because she seemed to have more mucus than normal. She started crying, and I was concerned they were hurting her. It was all I could do to refrain from making them stop. Right off the bat, I turned into this protective papa bear who wanted to come to her rescue and save her from harm.

The committed love you hold for your baby is unshakable, unconditional, and unfathomable. It is a blossoming hidden in the heart. It wells up and bursts forth at just the right moment. It is the foundation of fierce, fatherly love. This love springs from a deep well within and flows through you to your baby. Your baby awakens it and draws it from you. You become a brave warrior, capable of committing and offering your life. This is not small. This is huge.

CHAPTER 6

Unconditional love and absolute truth are two sides of the same coin—two expressions of one reality. From this perspective, absolute love is not just a feeling. It is an unconditional truth. In fact, committed love is the highest and most eloquent expression of truth. You build your relationship with your child upon the foundation of this truth. It represents a fullness that you are, but you do not contain it. The love you experience as father unites you to the potent, abundant mystery, and it is expressed through you.

If you already have a baby, you know exactly what this love is. If you have not yet had the experience, then all the volumes of words cannot adequately describe it. It is tangible, primal, transcendent, experiential, and transforming. It flows from you without effort when the moment is ripe.

THE OPPOSITE END OF THE CONTINUUM

There is danger in expectation. I do not want to mislead you. Not every man feels love for his baby immediately. If you do not immediately feel love for your baby, you need to know this is normal too. Respect your own experience, and don't make impossible demands on yourself to follow a script. Henry did not feel immediate love for his baby, and said:

I thought I would love my baby right away. But that's not how it worked for me. When I first saw the baby, I didn't feel much at all. If anything, I felt alienated, like this foreign person had just come into our lives. I feel guilty admitting this, because I love my son so much now, but in the early days I felt like this intruder had come into our lives and taken over. I resented the baby and his constant demands. And I had trouble connecting with him. I'll never forget the visit we made to another family who had a new baby and a three-year-old son. The babies got fussy and both women were occupied with them. That's when the boy turned to his father and asked, 'How long is Mom letting that baby stay here?' I laughed out loud when I heard him say that because I knew exactly how he felt.

A lot of men need time to recover from the shock of birth and all the changes and responsibilities that are suddenly dumped into their lives before they can warm up to the baby. If you are one of these men, respect your capacity and know you are not alone. If you respond like this father, know that most men pass through some form of this. It is part of the territory of becoming a father.

No one is immune from having to deal with their honest, valid, and conflicting emotions. Emotions are complex and powerful, and we do not always have a rational understanding of why we feel the way we do. People feel contradictory and opposing emotions all the time. You may love your baby (sometimes), but you may also find yourself resenting the intrusion. You may find yourself being overwhelmed by the unbelievable amount of sleep deprivation and work. You may feel like you are ignored, like your contribution is not valued. You may even experience grief as the reality settles in that your relationship and life have permanently altered.

Life changes so drastically after the birth of the first baby. Your identity changes. Your interests change. Your relationships change. There are a lot more demands. You have to cut out the fat. You may resent it. You purge on all levels. It takes time to get through it.

Everyone has to get through the best they can. Be compassionate toward yourself. Don't judge yourself. Navigate through how you have to. The more accepting you are of yourself, the more accepting you will be of your child as he or she grows.

CROSSING THE BARRIER

Every man needs markers to help him see the awakenings that are occurring as he prepares to be a father. One marker is the realization you could give your life to protect your child. Before the birth of your baby, it is likely you would hasten to leave a burning building, regarding your own life first. Instinct designs you for self-preservation. But after the birth of your child, it is likely you would willingly put yourself in harm's way to protect your child. Seth put it this way: *I would take a bullet for him.*

This shift crosses a major barrier. You are catapulted beyond the small self and are compelled to value another life over your own. When you realize you would risk your life to protect your child, you understand the magnitude of the transformations that are silently happening within as you prepare for this coming baby.

These awakenings occur when the time is ripe, in season. These shifts are not small and inconsequential. They are momentous and even a little mystical. They expand you beyond the edge of your small self, and reveal a glimpse of your greatness—so great you could give your life for another.

Fathering is an art that comes from a holy place. It is a rebirth on a higher level. Seekers practice for years in monastic traditions to get beyond the edge of their smallness, to expand into the greatness of being. If monks and adepts meditate for years to reach such a plane, fathers would do well to recognize their lofty height, and make good use of it.

While very few are called to risk their lives to save their children, most men willingly offer love, nourishment, and time. You discover your life by giving it away. Men minimize the summits to which they rise because they do not give themselves enough credit, and neither does anyone else, for the enormous offering they make in the work they do as father. Some men criticize themselves, and others may criticize them too, for their perceived shortcomings and not realize the vital contribution they are making to their families and society.

ENLIGHTENMENT

Enlightenment is always available. It is just so much more accessible in spaces like labor, birth, and becoming a father. Even though enlightenment is a fundamental attribute of birth, many are unaware of this remarkable truth. It's like holding a hidden gem you don't know you hold. How you perceive and experience birth is altered by uncovering and exposing this gem.

When we experience enlightenment, we relieve ourselves of what we think we are, but are not, to become more of the essential truth that we are. Enlightenment strips off the nonessential and simultaneously expands the essential—without limit. We encounter the truth that we are more than we realized. We move beyond our boundaries, and are drawn into a vast unexplored territory. The amazing thing isn't just that it expands our understanding of truth (truth and love emanate from the same source), but that we have the capacity to unite with it.

Being stripped of nonessentials and being expanded beyond limit is one of the great values of labor and birth. This stripping and expansion process is occurring for both the mother and the father. You have one foot on planet earth, and another in timelessness. The closer you are to the expanded reality, the closer you are to the truth of your own being.

PART TWO

GETTING READY: THE PREPARATION

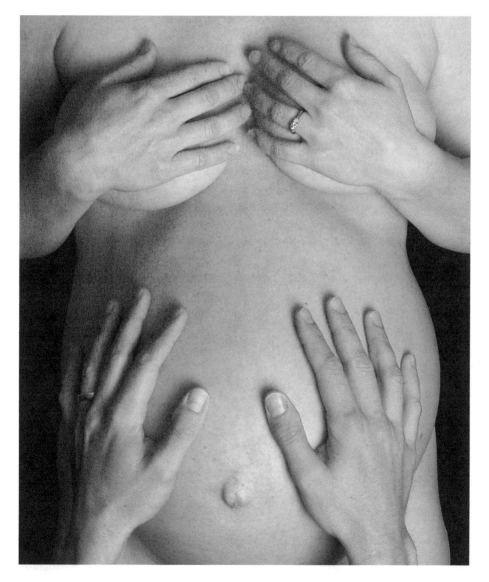

CHAPTER 7
BIRTH OPTIONS

WHERE WILL YOUR BABY BE BORN?

HOME BIRTHS
Home births are intimate and give couples control of their surroundings. If you and your partner choose to have a home birth, select a midwife or doctor who is experienced with them and supports your choice. An experienced practitioner provides medical expertise and screens the mother to make sure she is a good candidate for a home birth. Your practitioner will advise you on the supplementary supplies you need to gather. You and your partner also need to prepare and be well-informed on the process of birth.

Discuss a plan with your practitioner to access medical intervention, if necessary. Even though it is rare, if an emergency develops that cannot be dealt with in the home, having a plan to access sophisticated medical attention is wise. Couples who choose home births are actively involved in participating in their experience, are motivated in seeking out the necessary information, and are willing to do the additional preparation. Home births can be profoundly satisfying.

HOSPITAL BIRTHS
Some couples choose a hospital birth to ensure expert medical care is immediately available, if necessary. A few women have a medical condition that requires them to be in a hospital. Since some insurance companies only cover hospital births, finances may influence where your partner births. Some women want an epidural or want the option of choosing one. And some women have older children and want to recuperate an extra day or two before going back to a busy household; birthing centers are not set up for a long stay after birth.

Visit the hospitals covered by your policy; some hospitals are more user-friendly than others. Make sure your practitioner can practice in your selected hospital. Also, ask if your hospital routinely requires the use of IVs or electronic fetal monitors. If you want to use these interventions only if needed, some hospitals will waive their use with a doctor's order. Many couples have satisfying birth experiences in hospitals.

BIRTHING CENTERS

Birthing centers are smaller than hospitals and provide a homey atmosphere that accommodates the personal aspect of birthing. Explore the birthing center options in your community. Many birthing centers are run by nurse-midwives (CNM) who are highly skilled, professional, and experienced. Women who choose the birthing center option are medically screened by the midwife during pregnancy to ensure risks are minimized.

While birthing centers provide more intimacy and high-level care with less intervention, they are not equipped to handle some unexpected or emergency scenarios like cesarean birth. Many birthing centers are located near hospitals and are within easy reach of sophisticated medical attention, if needed. Drug choices are limited in birthing centers, and most women who birth in them are committed to doing labor without drugs. Your partner can be committed to doing labor without drugs in a hospital, but at a birthing center, an epidural is not an option. Birthing centers do not require IVs or fetal monitors, which gives the mother more autonomy and mobility during labor. Another advantage to a birthing center birth is that during labor, you are working with a midwife and staff who are present during the whole process. Labors are often shorter and there is less turbulence in the atmosphere. These aspects set a different tone to the quality of labor and contribute to making your birth experience more rewarding.

SCOPING OUT THE BATHTUB SCENE BEFORE LABOR

Once you and your partner decide where your baby will be born, check out the bathtub options. Some hospitals have jetted tubs in all rooms, but others have them only in a few rooms. Place an early request for a room with a tub, when appropriate. Taking a bath can soothe the mother and help labor progress with less discomfort. If you are having a home birth and do not have a large bathtub, consider acquiring a birth tub.

Barbara Harper, founder of the well established non-profit organization, Waterbirth International, advises: *Many women bring their own birth pool equipment with them to a hospital. Waterbirth International helps women advocate for the use of waterbirth immersion if their hospital does not allow them. Affordable birth pool kits for home or hospital use are also available.* To learn more about waterbirths or to acquire a tub, contact Waterbirth International at waterbirth.org.

GIVING BIRTH IN WATER

A waterbirth is an option for couples choosing a birthing center or a home birth. Since many hospitals have policies that prohibit waterbirths, you need to check with your individual hospital to determine whether a waterbirth is an option.

Here is Elizabeth's water-birth story:

We didn't plan on having a waterbirth. That's just how it played out. Shortly after arriving at the birth center, my labor got powerful and I panicked. That's when the midwife started running the water and got me into the tub. I relaxed in the water. My husband kept me warm and helped me to relax and focus on my breath between the contractions. Before long, I started grunting and growling and my body started pushing the baby out. It never occurred to me to get out of the water, and no one suggested it. The baby was really peaceful when she came out and the midwife reached down, pulled her from the water, and put her on my belly.

You do not need to be concerned about the baby taking his first breath underwater, because the baby will not breathe until exposed to air. Water encourages relaxation and waterbirths are often gentle for both mother and baby. Water gives the mother's perineum and abdominals support while pushing, which reduces or eliminates tearing. Babies born in water are often calmer at birth.

SHOULD WE USE A DOULA?

You and your partner also need to decide if you want to use a doula (a non-medical birth attendant specially trained to provide support during labor). There are benefits to using a skilled doula. She may shorten the time your partner labors, reduce or eliminate drug use, reduce or eliminate medical intervention, and make your experience more gratifying. A doula can also affect how labor progresses, how the couple responds to labor, the outcome of the birth, and how a couple feels about birth after it is over. This is a significant contribution since the birth of your child is a day you will always remember.

Some men want to be hands-on and active and are concerned about being upstaged or pushed aside by a doula. However, many men discover that using a doula supports them to be more confidently involved. Arthur shared his experience working with a doula: *Having a doula at the birth was good for us. She knew what was going on and what to do about it; the doula and I worked together as a team. My wife and I stayed connected. I think part of that was because the doula added a dynamic that kept our focus on track. She provided a lot of support and know-how for both of us.*

Insurance sometimes covers a portion of the doula expense, especially when connected to a hospital program. The disadvantage to using a hospital-staffed doula is that you do not choose who you work with or have an opportunity to develop a relationship with her prior to labor. You work with the doula that is currently scheduled.

The alternative is to hire a private doula. Advantages to using a private doula are that she is a valuable resource during pregnancy, and you develop a relationship with her before birth, which increases confidence levels. Some private doulas come to your home during early labor, and some come to your home postpartum to support the new mother.

Doulas provide experienced support and additional attention for the laboring woman and couple, but they are not trained to give medical advice or perform medical procedures. The medical staff is most concerned with the medical aspect of birth. Doulas are most concerned with providing support for the mother. Doulas and the medical staff have their separate level of work to do. Ideally they work together as a team and are not in competition with one another; they support one another. A professional birth assistant's role is to help the mother have the most satisfying birth possible; to support the couple to do birth the way they choose rather than impose a personal agenda; to maintain a professional demeanor with staff members and other attendants; and to provide continual care for the mother and family during the entire process.

Your partner may not want to use a doula. If you and your partner decide to work alone as a couple, you will be more successful if you prepare. This book is designed to prepare you so you can make a difference for your partner whether or not you use a doula.

Since the mother has an innate knowledge of what is right for her, it is wise to leave the bulk of the decision regarding using a doula to your partner. Whether you use one or not, your role is critical.

WHAT ABOUT HAVING OTHER ATTENDANTS?

Your partner may want her mother, sister, a close friend, or a massage therapist with her. In a few instances, the woman's mother, mother-in-law, father, sister, sister-in-law, older children, and close friends all come for the birth. There can be a place for everyone's involvement. However, since birth is such a personal and intimate event, it is wise to restrict extra people to those with whom your partner has a deep emotional connection and professional attendants who have a purpose for being there.

When I attend births with people other than the father, I enlist their assistance. They can assist the mother to change positions, press on pressure points during contractions, and massage the mother. They can also get drinks, extra pillows, ice or hot packs, run bath water, get the shower ready, etc. A few extra hands minimize extraneous work so you can stay at your partner's side. No matter who comes to the birth, everyone's focus needs to remain centered on the laboring woman, and you need to be the one who remains at your partner's side.

Occasionally in a long labor, if there are several people in attendance, a few of them gather in a corner and talk. The laboring mother often finds this distracting or upsetting. Sometimes people want to eat while in the room. The smell of food may nauseate your partner. It is your job to attend and support your partner, and to ensure the environment is peaceful and conducive to the work she needs to do. This may require you to take the role of the stern father to diminish disruptions. You may need to send people out of the room temporarily to eat or talk. Occasionally, you may need to close the door and let them know they are not to disturb you until you call them in.

If you and your partner have older children, discuss the option of having them attend the birth. Jo Anne shared her experience of having her older children attend the birth:

I wanted our two older children to attend our birth. However, I did not want them present during labor. I wanted that time to be exclu-

sively for my husband and me. Our children stayed in the lounge and played board games while I labored. Once I was pushing, my husband called them to watch the birth of their sister. Immediately after she was born I held her, and our whole family gathered around her. There was this circle of loving faces gazing upon her. It felt complete for us to be together to greet her in the first moments of her life. My older children bonded with the baby immediately, and the baby's transition into their lives was easy for them.

Each family makes its own decision based on the mother's desire and the ages and temperaments of the children. Sibling classes are available for older children to prepare them for birth, or you and your partner may choose to do the preparation. However, your partner may not want her older children at the birth. She may need privacy, or she may feel it would be upsetting to her or the children. Support her in her choice.

CHAPTER 8
COMMONLY USED LABOR TERMS

UNDERSTANDING COMMONLY USED TERMS
EFFACEMENT AND DILATION OF THE CERVIX

The *cervix* is the opening (mouth) of the uterus. The end of the tunnel-shaped vagina is attached to it. The average pregnant cervix is three to four centimeters long, or about 1¼ inches. During labor, the cervix must thin and open. Thinning of the cervix is called *effacement*. Opening of the cervix is called *dilatation.*

During effacement, the cervix softens, rounds, thins, and flattens. If the cervix is 50 percent effaced, the cervix has rounded and thinned to two centimeters in length. If the cervix is 75 percent effaced, it has thinned to one centimeter in length. If the cervix is 100 percent effaced, it has completely flattened and thinned. Besides effacing 100 percent, the cervix must dilate to ten centimeters wide, or about four inches. The purpose of contractions is twofold. They work to completely efface and dilate the cervix. They also work to push the baby out of the uterus, through the birth canal, and into the world.

Toward the end of pregnancy, hormones and prostaglandins ripen (soften) the cervix and change its angle. Early in pregnancy, the cervix angles toward your partner's back and feels firm, like the tip of the nose. In preparation for birth, the cervix angles to a more forward position, and feels soft like a puckered mouth.

You may have felt some of the changes in your partner's cervix while making love. Sexual intercourse is beneficial during a normal pregnancy because orgasm tones the uterus and releases endorphins and oxytocin, which increase well-being. Because semen contains prostaglandins, making love is healthy for the cervix. If you and your partner have concerns, consult your medical caretaker.

It is not uncommon for a woman's cervix to begin to efface and dilate weeks or days before labor begins. On rare occasions, the cervix fully effaces before labor begins. Other women do no effacing or dilating until the onset of labor. The cervix must be 100 percent effaced and ten centimeters dilated before the baby can move out of the womb, through the opening of the cervix, and into the birth canal (vagina). From this perspective, you can easily understand how one purpose of contraction is expansion, opening.

If your partner comes home from a checkup with the news that she is 75 percent effaced and two centimeters dilated, you will know what she is talking about. This news means that your partner's cervix has thinned to about one centimeter in length and has opened to two centimeters wide. Once your partner has started effacing and dilating, the baby can come at any time, but it still may be days or weeks away. Even if your partner has done no effacing or dilating, labor can start at any time once the pregnancy is full-term and she is ripe, meaning the cervix has softened and is in position for birth.

MUCUS PLUG

During pregnancy, a *mucus plug* forms along the length of the cervix. While some women lose the mucus plug days or weeks before the onset of labor with no other consequences, others pass the mucus plug in labor. It may also come out in stages. Your partner may pass thick strands of blood or brownish-tinged hard mucus in late pregnancy, or she may have a *bloody show* during labor, accompanied by blood-tinged mucus.

PLACENTA AND AMNIOTIC SAC

The *placenta* is a large, disc-shaped, meaty organ attached to the inside wall of the uterus. Its function is to provide the baby with nourishment and oxygen and remove wastes. The baby is attached to the placenta by his *umbilical cord*; oxygen and nourishment travel from the placenta through the umbilical cord to the baby. The baby's wastes also travel through the umbilical cord to the placenta for removal.

The baby and the umbilical cord are surrounded by the fluid-filled *amniotic sac* (bag of waters) for protection. One purpose of the amniotic sac is to prevent outside bacteria from getting to the baby. If your partner leaks water before labor begins, she needs to alert her medical caretaker promptly. Amniotic fluid is clear; if the water is green-brown tinged or has a fetid odor, let the medical caretaker know immediately.

The amniotic sac can rupture (break or tear) and begin to leak at any time during labor. If the amniotic sac ruptures with a gush, labor may move rapidly; contact your medical caretaker promptly. Vomiting, coughing, or sneezing, may cause the amniotic sac to break during labor. It can also break spontaneously from the pressure of contractions. Lilly shared her experience of her water breaking in early labor: *After using the bathroom, I felt warm water running down my leg. For a while I thought I was leaking urine, but then I realized my water had broken.*

Once the amniotic sac has ruptured in labor, there is more pressure on the baby's head and the contractions are generally more intense. Artificially rupturing the sac as an intervention to increase the tempo of labor may cause the cord to compress and restrict oxygen to the baby. It is wise to allow the sac to rupture on its own without intervention.

BRAXTON-HICKS CONTRACTIONS AND PRELABOR

In the months before labor begins, your partner may feel periodic, intermittent *Braxton-Hicks contractions.* These contractions are like tension-and-release exercises that tone the uterus, but they do not efface or dilate the cervix. If you place your hand on your partner's abdomen during a Braxton-Hicks contraction, you can feel her uterus harden. Some women experience these contractions frequently, and some women rarely notice them.

In the weeks and days before the onset of labor, your partner may experience an increase of pressure, contractions, and rhythmic waves called *prelabor*. Prelabor is also called *false labor* because the waves are not persistent and stop after a few hours. However, these contractions are not really false labor because they begin the process of thinning and opening the cervix. Juliana experienced them in her second pregnancy: *I was having these waves that got really strong for a few hours before they petered out. It went on for days. I went for a checkup and I was 90 percent effaced and three centimeters dilated. Once labor started, it took three hours for the baby to be born.*

TIMING CONTRACTIONS

Once labor begins, time contractions periodically. However, keep in mind that for centuries women have delivered babies without timing contractions. Don't be obsessed with timing. It distracts your partner from easing into labor and may make her anxious, which further slows the process. Remember: mere observation can alter an event. Early in labor, observe your partner's behavior and note occasionally how close her waves are coming without drawing much attention to it.

Once contractions are making obvious progress, record the pattern. To time contractions, you need a watch with a second hand or a stopwatch. Time the frequency and length of at least five consecutive contractions to establish a pattern. For example, if your partner has a contraction at 7:05, the next at 7:15, and the next at 7:25, and this pattern continues for five or more contractions, your partner's contractions are ten minutes apart. Ten minutes is the interval between contractions—from the beginning of one contraction to the beginning of the next.

Use the second hand to time the length as well. If the contraction starts at 7:05 and lasts thirty-five seconds, the length of the contraction is thirty-five seconds. If the next wave starts at 7:15 and lasts for thirty-five seconds, and this pattern continues for five consecutive contractions, the length of the contractions is thirty-five seconds.

Besides the frequency and length, note the intensity. Observe your partner's behavior both during and between the contractions. Is she able to talk during the contraction? Is she grimacing? Is the contraction drawing her in and commanding all of her attention? Is she spacey? Is she able to come out of the contraction and be in charge of what is going on around her, or is she no longer social between contractions? Make a note. Now you have an idea of how strong the contractions are—the intensity.

Once labor is making obvious progress, you get so drawn into attending your partner you won't have time to track five consecutive waves. Periodically, make a mental note of how fast the waves are coming. To chart the progression of several rounds of five consecutive contractions during early labor, follow the example on the next page:

Time	Length	Frequency: Interval	Intensity: Behavior and Symptoms (such as social interaction, focus, grimacing, nausea, or vaginal discharge)
3:17 p.m.	45 sec.		Walking; starting to focus during contraction, but talking in between
3:24 p.m.	45 sec.	7-min. interval	Frequent trips to the bathroom
3:31 p.m.	45 sec.	7-min.	Less social
3:38 p.m.	47 sec.	7-min.	Wants pressure on her lower back and is focus-ing with contraction
3:44 p.m.	50 sec.	6-min.	Talking in between contractions, but not during them
3:50 p.m.	50 sec.	6-min.	Is starting to grimace during contraction

THE BABY'S POSITION

When your partner begins labor, your baby is most commonly in a head-down position. If the back of the head is facing the mother's belly, this position is called *occiput anterior*. Anterior position is op-timal for mother and baby. A baby in anterior position initially pres-ents facedown as it emerges out of the birth canal.

About 25 percent of the time, the back of the baby's head is facing the mother's back. This position is called *occiput posterior*. A mother whose baby is in posterior position experiences more back pressure and usually needs firm counterpressure on her lower back. All-fours positions can relieve some back pressure and may help the baby ro-tate into an anterior position before birth. But not all babies do so. A posterior baby initially presents faceup as it emerges. The attend-ing nurse may make a good-natured joke about the baby being born sunny-side up.

EPISIOTOMY

An *episiotomy* is a surgical incision that increases the diameter of the vaginal opening to accommodate the emergence of the baby's head. The practitioner uses scissors to make a cut from the lower part of the vaginal opening through the perineum tissue toward the rectum. An episiotomy is a precautionary, preemptive move to prevent tearing of the perineum as some practitioners feel it is easier to repair an incision than a tear. But there is no guarantee there will be no additional tearing.

Discuss with your medical practitioners their views on and use of episiotomies. You want a practitioner who does not routinely perform episiotomies; who supports the perineum after the baby crowns; and who allows the baby's head to emerge at its own pace, which helps to reduce or eliminate tearing. This approach sometimes prevents a woman from doing any tearing.

I know this next example sounds strange, but think of the difference between cutting and tearing lettuce to make a salad. A torn leaf of lettuce tears along natural lines. Cutting the lettuce is a more rigid way. A tear can be less damaging to the perineal tissue than an incision because it occurs along natural lines.

An episiotomy may be performed if the baby is in distress and needs to be delivered immediately; if forceps are used in the delivery; to prevent tearing of the rectum or labia (internal lips on the exterior of the vaginal opening); or if the woman's perineum is unyielding, and she has trouble pushing the baby out.

If an episiotomy is performed, the practitioner may not use a local anesthetic. The episiotomy feels like a pinch. Because there is tremendous pressure in the birth canal from the baby's head, the mother may feel some relief from the pressure after it is performed. The incision varies in length, depending on the situation and the judgment of the attending practitioner. Episiotomies used to be given routinely in hospital births, but have now fallen into disfavor and criticism. It is wise to request that no episiotomy be performed, unless there is a medical reason that warrants one.

INTRAVENOUS FLUIDS AND FETAL MONITORS

The purpose of *intravenous fluid (IV)* is to keep the woman's body hydrated during labor. IVs are also used to administer some drugs, if needed. The purpose of the *electronic fetal monitor (EFM)* is to track and record the baby's heart rate, as well as the frequency, duration, and intensity of the contractions. Birthing centers do not administer IVs or use EFMs as standard procedure, and of course, they are not used in a home birth.

Hospitals however, administer IVs and use EFMs routinely. If your partner is having a hospital birth and is opposed to using either of these, discuss it with your medical practitioner before labor. If her practitioner agrees there are no medical reasons that warrant their use, he or she will often waive one or both of these.

When no IV or EFM is used, your partner has freer mobility during labor. Fluid levels are maintained by sipping drinks. Contractions are monitored by timing them. The baby's heart rate is monitored by periodic use of a stethoscope or an ultrasound fetoscope, which is considered adequate for an uncomplicated birth. Listening to the heartbeat also provides personal attention for your partner on a regular basis.

If your partner decides to use an IV, or if there is a medical reason that makes it necessary to use one, your job is to make sure the IV fluid bag is hung from an IV mobile stand and not hung on the IV pole attached to the bed. An IV stand with wheels is essential for your partner's mobility. When your partner wants to walk, push the IV stand along with her.

If your partner decides to use an EFM, or if there is a medical reason that makes it necessary to use one, the staff wraps a wide fabric band—held in place by Velcro—around your partner's abdomen. In it is secured an ultrasound device strategically positioned to track the baby's heart rate. The device has two wires connected to the electronic fetal monitor machine. One records contractions; the other records the baby's heart rate.

When your partner wants to move farther than the wires allow, leave the Velcro belt with the ultrasound device in place on her abdomen and detach the wires from the machine. Tuck the wires into the Velcro band to keep them from hanging. If the band comes off in the maneuvering, leave it. The nurse will rewrap the band and reposition the ultrasound device when your partner returns.

When your partner returns, plug the wires back into the machine. The ends of the wires are marked so they are easy to match. If you reattach the wires and the machine does not pick up the heart rate, the nurse will come and reposition the ultrasound device. If this sounds a little daunting, have the staff help you with it the first time or two. Once you get it, it's straightforward.

One downside to an EFM is a couple can get too involved in watching it. The woman may focus her attention on the external monitor instead of focusing within. The man may get sidetracked by watching the fetal monitor instead of focusing on his partner. Monitor yourself and don't allow the EFM to distract you from your partner.

Some practitioners use an internal application that is attached to the baby's head. This requires rupturing the amniotic sac, is invasive, and increases complications and risk. Avoid internal monitoring. A newer, wireless model, called a telemetry monitor is available in some hospitals. Inquire if your hospital has one, and request they use the telemetry if your partner uses a fetal monitor.

CHAPTER 9

THE MAP: THE THREE STAGES OF LABOR

1. **Stage I: Dilation**—This stage is divided into three phases: Early, Active, and Transition Labor. The purpose of the first stage is to completely efface and dilate the cervix to ten centimeters, so the baby can move out of the womb and into the birth canal. During the dilation stage, dramatic changes occur. Your partner changes from a person you know into a woman totally absorbed and overtaken by labor. Early labor is generally manageable, but active and transition labor demand your partner's entire energy.

2. **Stage II: Pushing and Birth**—The purpose of the second stage of labor is birth. This is the pushing phase, also known as the *descent* stage. The baby descends out of the womb and through the birth canal, and is born. This is a dynamic stage. Your partner comes out of the consuming labor trance and becomes more alert. She focuses her energy to do this most important and holy work—birth the baby.

3. **Stage III: Delivery of the Placenta**—The purpose of the third stage is to deliver the placenta, also called the *placental* stage. The placenta is referred to as the *afterbirth*. During this stage, you and your partner will be entranced by your new baby and relieved that labor is behind you. Hold your baby during this period and immerse yourself in the experience.

While there are common markers in the progression of labor, each woman's labor is unique and distinct. Typical characteristics of each stage of labor are described below, for easy reference:

FIRST STAGE OF LABOR: DILATION is the opening of the cervix to ten centimeters. The first stage of labor is divided into three phases: early, active, and transition.

1. EARLY LABOR PHASE

*   Cervix dilates to four centimeters.

- Early labor lasts from one to twelve hours (or longer).
- Contractions often start out vague and slow, with long intervals between them. Early contractions last ten to fifteen seconds and occur at fifteen-to twenty-minute intervals. The mother is able to talk and tend to other tasks besides labor. Many women continue whatever activities they are involved in until contractions start demanding their attention.
- Contractions get progressively more rhythmic, stronger, longer, and closer together until they become thirty to fifty seconds long and occur at seven- to ten-minute intervals. Time contractions periodically.
- Once contractions are progressing, encourage the mother to focus. Don't talk to her during a contraction. Minimize distractions. Generally, as early labor progresses, your partner gets more drawn into labor, is less social, and needs to concentrate during her contraction.
- Offer fluids. Her body needs to be hydrated to sustain labor.
- She needs your companionship and loving attention.
- If your partner's amniotic sac breaks with a gush during early labor, she is likely to move rapidly into active labor. Contact her practitioner and observe her behavior.

2. **ACTIVE LABOR PHASE**
   - Cervix dilates four to eight centimeters. This phase lasts one to six hours or longer.
   - The interval between contractions gets shorter and the contractions get longer and more intense. Time contractions periodically.
   - This is the phase in which you and your partner move to the birth facility, unless you are doing a home birth.
   - Medical caretakers may recommend going to the birth facility when contractions are sixty seconds long and five minutes apart; however, individual instructions vary. Be sure to check with your medical caretaker. If you are having a home birth, your caretaker needs to be notified by this point, unless she has already arrived.
   - As active labor progresses, contractions demand all of your partner's attention and resources both during and in between

the waves. Minimize distractions. Nothing else matters but labor.

- Talking becomes difficult, and she only speaks when necessary.
- Your partner enters an altered state. Her rational mind shuts down. She has no sense of time.
- It is difficult for her to process external information. When you communicate with her, get within a six-to twelve-inch radius of her face.
- By this stage, you will no longer be timing contractions, but will make a periodic mental note that contractions are three minutes apart, etc.
- You will use your skills to help her breath remain fluid and flowing.
- She needs you to help her change positions periodically.
- She needs your exclusive attention and protection.

3. **TRANSITION LABOR PHASE**
   - Cervix dilates eight to ten centimeters. (*see* **Figure 9.1**)
   - This is the shortest phase, but the most intense. It lasts from fifteen to ninety minutes or longer.
   - Contractions last ninety seconds to two minutes (or longer) and occur at thirty-second intervals (more or less).
   - Contractions can be almost continual, with only a small break in between.
   - Your partner can speak, if at all, only with great effort.
   - She may feel like she cannot continue. She may have no clue (and neither may anyone else) that she is nearing the end of the first stage of labor. She may weep. She may vomit. She may drop off to sleep between the waves of labor. She may demand drugs.
   - She needs your assurance and rock-solid mountain stability.
   - However, some women remain completely focused through transition labor. Tracking the frequency of contractions and observing how intently your partner needs to focus are clues to help you determine whether she is in transition.
   - Toward the end of transition, the mother feels pressure as the baby's head begins to press toward the birth canal. This is accompanied by an urge to push.

- At the end of transition, her demeanor changes. She is more able to talk, more responsive, and more aware of her surroundings.
- An internal examination is performed to make sure the cervix has completely dilated to ten centimeters, and she is ready to push.
- This phase is intense, and she needs you to be completely there for her.

SECOND STAGE OF LABOR: PUSHING AND BIRTHING is the stage where the baby descends out of the uterus, through the cervix, and into the birth canal, and then is born.

- Your partner experiences an overwhelming urge to push (or not). She may involuntarily push with contractions.
- This phase lasts twenty minutes to three hours (or longer).
- Contractions last sixty to ninety seconds (or more) and become two to five minutes apart, giving your partner time to rest from the vigorous work of pushing.
- Your partner feels tremendous pressure as the baby moves down the birth canal.
- Your partner's behavior changes. She can talk and communicate with the external world. She may feel exhilarated.
- She needs you to help her get into an optimal pushing position.
- She may need you to help support her position while she pushes.
- You may see her as supremely powerful and determined while she pushes.
- For some women, pushing is a colossal endeavor. The mother may become exhausted or discouraged. She needs your encouragement and unconditional support.
- For other women, pushing is straightforward, and the birth is quick.
- The baby crowns when the head presses against the perineum (tissue between the vagina and the anus), bulging the perineum. The medical caretaker supports the perineum. This is a period of intense stretching of perineal tissue, and it may hurt or burn. This is also the time that an episiotomy is performed, only if necessary.

- The baby's head emerges. The baby rotates. A shoulder emerges. The other shoulder emerges, and the baby slides out. Your baby is born. You may want to catch your baby and be the one who gives your baby to your partner.
- Your partner wants you there to share the birth. This is an intimate time of sharing as you both welcome your baby into the world and begin the bonding process. (*see* **Figures 9.1 and 9.2**)

THIRD STAGE OF LABOR: DELIVERY OF THE PLACENTA

After birth, the uterus continues contracting and clamping down, in an effort to completely detach the placenta from the uterine wall.

- The baby's umbilical cord is clamped and cut, which completely separates the baby from the mother's body. It is wise to wait until the umbilical cord has stopped pulsating before clamping and cutting it. You may want to cut the cord.
- The placenta is expelled from the uterus around seven to twenty (or more) minutes after birth, often with a gush of blood and fluid. When the placenta slides out, the mother is often so entranced with her baby that she barely notices.
- The placenta usually detaches without intervening assistance; however, your partner may be asked to push to assist in the delivery the placenta and an attendant may massage her abdomen to stimulate the uterus to contract.
- The placenta is thoroughly examined by the medical practitioner to make sure all of it has passed.
- Her perineum is examined and repaired, if needed. A local anesthetic is administered through a shot directly into the perineum if your partner needs stitches. But this rarely disturbs her; her attention is focused on the baby.
- Mother and baby need to stay warm.
- Due to hormone changes, the mother may shake or tremble.
- The uterus continues contracting. Occasionally, a mother who has had previous births experiences the contractions or afterpains of the uterus as painful. You may need to use your skills to assist her with the pain.
- Your partner will likely be holding or nursing your baby during the placental stage. You can hold the baby during this stage too. Tell the mother what a great job she did.

CHAPTER 9

The above description of the stages of labor is a guide. How labor develops and what different women experience varies. The interval and length of contractions varies widely, especially during early labor. While some experts define transition labor as seven to ten centimeters, others define it as eight to ten. Because it is unwise to administer pain relief medication too late in labor, I have defined transition labor as eight to ten centimeters, however every woman and every birth are unique and distinct.

HOW LONG WILL LABOR LAST?

A normal labor lasts anywhere from two to twenty-four hours (or more). An average first-time labor lasts twelve to seventeen hours. But don't take this time frame literally. Lots of first-time births are shorter and some are longer. Each successive labor is generally shorter and easier, but not necessarily. There is no way to predict how long your partner's labor will last. There are always surprises.

INTERNAL EXAMS: DON'T PUT TOO MUCH EMPHASIS ON DILATION

During labor, the staff performs periodic internal exams to check the effacement and dilation of the cervix, as well as the baby's station (location of the baby within the mother's pelvis). Even though it is tempting, don't put too much emphasis on the dilation measurement. Judge progress by your partner's behavior, as well as the frequency, length, and intensity of the contractions. If you use dilation as a gauge, your partner can get discouraged if labor does not seem to be progressing. This will sabotage her concentration and confidence to get through labor.

Here is Paula's story:

I had been in serious, mind-bending labor for what seemed like forever. When the nurse checked me, she told me I was only at six centimeters. I can't tell you how discouraged I was. I wanted to cry. I remember thinking, 'If it's this bad now, I'll never make it. I can't do it. I want drugs.' But my husband started a five-to-one countdown with me (See Chapter 10 for description). I managed to get through the next five waves. Then he talked me into five more, and then five more. He kept counting until the waves were so intense, I couldn't talk. My husband told me he suspected I was in transition labor because my contractions were practically on top of each other. Then I got an urge to push. My husband went to tell the nurse I was pushing, and she didn't believe I could possibly be pushing. But I was.

Dilation is not an accurate gauge to determine the length of labor, and nurses may not always be accurate in their measurement. Women can seemingly make no progress, not dilating for a few hours—and then dilate rapidly during the next hour. Be your partner's mountain and remain stable, no matter what the external situation appears to be.

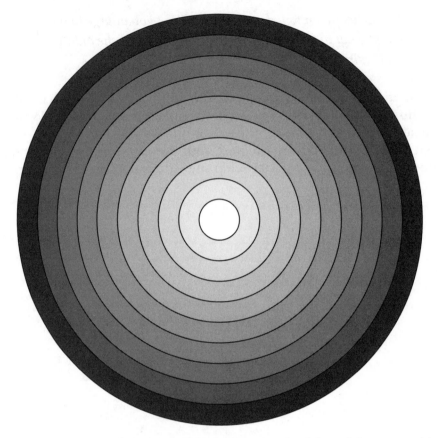

Figure 9.1 Dilation Chart: Early labor, 0-4 cm; active labor, 4-8 cm; transition labor, 8-10 cm. Ten centimeters is also referred to as dilated to "five fingers" (a finger's width equals 2 cm).

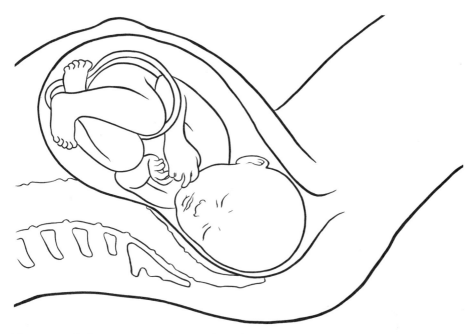

Figure 9.2 Dilation is complete and pushing phase begins.

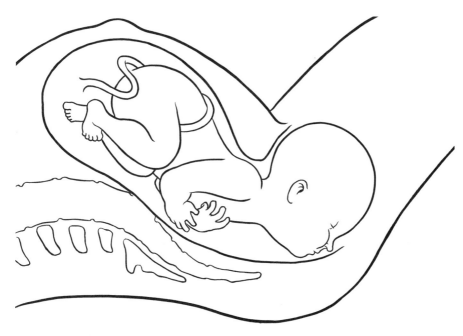

Figure 9.3 Baby's head emerges from the birth canal.

CHAPTER 10

HOW TO USE BREATH AND OTHER TOOLS DURING LABOR

This chapter and the next offer several tools, strategies, techniques, and focal points to assist your partner during labor. These strategies help your partner focus, cope with pain, and relax during labor. Observe how your partner responds. As her needs change, you will use different strategies. Even though these two chapters detail how to use the breath and focal points, do not underestimate the value of helping your partner change positions periodically. (*See* Chapter 16 for details on positions you and your partner can use during labor.)

NOSTRIL BREATHING

Your partner will use nostril breathing during early labor, but once labor becomes active, she will likely inhale through the nose and exhale through the mouth. Nostrils are designed to filter, warm, and moisturize air before it reaches the lungs. During nostril breathing, air flows through the nasal turbinates. Nasal turbinates increase the velocity of air and stimulate nerve endings, which positively affect brain function and the mind-body system.

Inhaling through the mouth uses more energy, bypasses the important stimulation of nerve endings in the nostrils, and is dehydrating. Since conserving your partner's energy and keeping her hydrated are important, nostril breathing is preferred. Inhaling through the mouth stimulates the upper lobes of the lungs, which then cue the nervous system to release fight, fright, or flight responses. Since the nervous system and your partner's sense of well-being are intimately connected to breath, inhaling through the nose helps the mother travel through labor with less distress. Use a decongestant spray to unclog your partner's nasal passages if she gets congested.

There are exceptions to nostril breathing. When you talk or sound (described later), you exhale through the mouth. When you yawn or cough, you inhale and exhale through the mouth. The idea is to breathe through the nose when practical. Don't be rigid. Make room for exceptions.

USE SOFT GAZING AND SIMPLE BREATH AWARENESS

Your goal is to have a continual peripheral awareness of the quality of your partner's breath. The best way to be aware of your partner's breathing is to apply the *soft gazing technique*. To use soft gazing, relax your eyes, unrestrict your breath, and take in your partner's breath pattern with a soft, wide-open gaze. If you cannot detect how she is breathing, tune in and breathe with her. There will be times when you are exclusively focused on your partner's breathing. But this is not a prescription to hover over her breath; that will irritate her.

Encourage your partner to let her breath flow. Your partner focuses on the breath both during the waves and between the waves. Simple breath awareness helps your partner relax. Use this technique until it no longer works.

BREATH IS AN INSTANT CLUE AS TO HOW YOUR PARTNER IS COPING

By observing breath, you monitor how your partner is coping with labor. Her breath pattern will cue you as to when she needs assistance. If her breath remains fluid and flowing, she is managing. If her breath becomes erratic, rapid, shallow, or exhibits long pauses, she needs assistance. Jack, a man with whom I worked, commented on how easy it was for him to use the breath as a gauge to determine how his partner was managing labor: *I finally put it together that observing my wife's breathing was an instant clue as to when she needed help. Once I got that, I didn't have to keep asking her how she was doing. And I didn't feel so anxious about when to help her. I could just tell by the breath. It was so much easier to use breath as a sign as to when I needed to step in and help.*

If your partner's breath becomes choppy or exhibits long pauses, she is using breath to *fight* the waves by pitting her strength against the force of contractions. Choppy breath with punctuated pauses increases pain and depletes her energy on unproductive maneuvers to manage labor. If her breath rises to the upper chest and is rapid and shallow or if she hyperventilates, she is using breath to *run away* from the rising force of contractions. If she runs, she gets caught in the centrifugal force (remember the hurricane image) and labor is more painful.

If your partner exhibits either of these breath patterns, she needs your intervening assistance. When your partner uses the breath to fight or run from labor, her diaphragm becomes rigid, which creates tension in the whole body and increases pain. If you help her focus on breath and encourage her to let her breath flow, it helps her to un-restrict the diaphragm and allows breath to move more fluidly, which diminishes tension and pain. Breath also gives her a focus and a place to ground herself in the body. Below are details on how to assist your partner to use a more effective breath pattern.

HAND-ON-UPPER-ABDOMEN TECHNIQUE™

To intervene and assist your partner to find a more effective breath pattern, use *hand-on-upper-abdomen technique™*. To use this tech-nique, place your hand on her upper abdomen between her lower ribs and navel. Your warm hand on her soft upper abdomen, above her contracting uterus, gives her a place to center her attention.

Do not press too hard, but press firmly enough to give her a focus for where to bring her breath. Get close to her and say: *Breathe into my hand.* Her goal is make your hand rise with the inhalation and fall with the exhalation. If she cannot find the way to a more effec-tive breath pattern say: *Make my hand move with the inhalation.* At the same time, apply slightly more pressure on her soft upper abdomen to help guide her breath to your hand.

Your goal is to help her use the breath to relax the diaphragm so that it finds a more natural flowing rhythm. The hand-on-upper-ab-domen technique may take you and your partner a few waves to es-tablish. Be gentle, but be persistent. She may want you to leave your hand in place because your warm hand stabilizes her and gives her a focal point to breathe into during the wave. Cue in to her comfort and adjust the pressure of your hand accordingly.

There may be times when your hand disturbs her during the wave. When that happens, remove your hand. Go with her specific comfort level, which is always changing. You can continue to cue her with hand-on-upper-abdomen technique between the waves and re-mind her: *Breathe here.* You can also cue her with the phrase: *Let your breath flow like the surf of the ocean.* This gives her an idea to work with. Placing your hand on her upper abdomen provides great assistance. It gives her a focus and helps her to consciously use breath to reduce anxiety, tension, and pain.

CHAPTER 10

SOUNDING TECHNIQUE

When breathing into your hand ceases to work, try *sounding technique* with the exhalation. This technique has a physiological basis in that sounding helps to regulate the breathing. It elongates the exhalation and frees the diaphragm, which relaxes the whole body. Make a low sound—*aaahhhhh*—near her ear. Make the sound to get her going and encourage her to say *aaahhhhh* with you. Let her find her own sound and her own rhythm. The idea is to connect the pain to the sound and groan it out. I have attended labors where we sounded together through most of late active and transition labor. This technique can be extremely effective.

If you are comfortable doing it, sound with her. This comes naturally to some, as we have the desire to enter into another's sphere to support them. Say: *Good job. Move the pain out with the sound.*

Women often get into a rhythm with sounding, and it becomes a ritual, which is soothing and focusing. The long exhalation unrestricts the diaphragm and relaxes her body, and the sound gives her a focal point. Many women feel they are actually moving the pain out with the breath and the vibration of the sound. The inhalation naturally rises after spending the exhalation in sound, and the breath takes on a healthier rhythm.

Each mother finds her own sound, which can be roaring and primal, or it may be subdued, more like a sigh, depending on the mother and where she is in labor. By connecting the pain to the exhalation and sound, she gets the breath flowing with her labor instead of using it to resist or run away. She diminishes pain as she relaxes her body and creates a focus.

Your partner may be silent or make subdued sounds between the waves. **Encourage her to let the end of the wave wash away with a sighing exhalation.** Be aware of your own breathing and comfort. Offer fluids. Let her rest.

TENSION LEVELS AND VOICE PITCH

Low-pitched sounds help your partner release tension and flow with labor. Groans, moans, sighs, primal sounds, and roars are good sounds in labor. Your partner can be as loud or as quiet in sounding as she wants, but if the pitch of her voice gets high, tension increases. If she makes *eeeeee* sounds, if she screeches or shrieks, she is in distress. Assist her by making a low-pitched *aaahhhhh* or *mmmmmmm* sound directly into her ear, so it is the predominant sound she hears. Hearing a low sound helps her to drop the pitch of her voice and calm herself.

Observe any parent in any culture pick up an infant in distress, and the parent will often instinctively use low-pitched sounds near the baby's ear to soothe the infant. These lower sounds are ancient, universal, and hardwired into us.

MONITOR FACIAL TENSION: USE A TOUCH-AND-SAY™

Besides monitoring breath and voice pitch, you need to monitor tension levels in your partner's face. The face is the window to the body. If the face is tense, the body is tense. If the face is relaxed, the body is relaxed. You do not have time to monitor your partner's body between the waves of labor, but you do have time to monitor the face.

The eye is the single most important facial feature because it is a powerful shortcut for the whole body. When the mother's eye softens, her whole body softens. If her eye remains tense between the waves of labor, lightly stroke the bone near her eye while saying: *Soften your eye*. It is important to combine touch with simultaneous clear verbal instruction—a *touch-and-say*™.

This makes your message clear and concise because you are using two neural paths of communication, which makes it easier for the mother to grasp your meaning. In deep labor, she is in an altered state, and you want to spare her the wasted energy of trying to figure out what you are doing or saying.

Monica shared: *My husband stroked my eye and I couldn't figure out what he was doing. Then he said, 'Relax your eye,' and I thought, 'What is he talking about? My eye? Where is my eye?' I finally relaxed my eye, but it took a lot of effort to figure it out.*

A touch-and-say spares your partner from spending her energy trying to figure out what you are doing or saying. It is not your job to *make* her relax. If she does not relax, it is because she cannot. After you have pointed out the tension, your job is done. Leave it be for now.

MONITOR THE JAW AND MOUTH

Another area of the face that is important to monitor is the jaw area, which includes the mouth and tongue. In ancient maps of the face, the jaw corresponds to the pelvis and hip joints. The tongue corresponds to the sacral area. The mouth corresponds to the pelvic floor and cervix. If her mouth is tight, she is unconsciously using her energy to resist opening at her cervix. Since the point of labor is to open the cervix, assist her to keep her mouth soft. Use a touch-and-say: stroke the corner of her mouth, and simultaneously say: *Soften your mouth.*

Many women clench their jaw during labor. Women clench in an effort to hang on and brace themselves against the force of labor. If your partner clenches her jaw, stroke it and say: *Soften your jaw.* Encouraging her to make the *aaahhhhh* sound is particularly helpful because it opens the mouth and releases the jaw and tongue. I have worked with clients who were habitual jaw-clenchers and we *aaahhh-hh*ed together through their entire labor to keep the jaw unclenched. It became a ritual and they found the repetition and vibration of the sound to be centering and soothing.

Andrea shared her experience of using sound to release her jaw: *Once active labor kicked in, I started bracing myself against the contractions. I tensed up, and it was like I was afraid to let go. I didn't even know it, but I was biting down and clenching my jaw. My husband got me going with the aaahhhhh sound, and I didn't stop until I started pushing. I don't think I could have gotten through labor without drugs if he hadn't gotten me sounding. It was the one thing that really helped.*

CHOOSE ONE AREA AT A TIME

Between contractions, give the mother one focus at a time so she does not get overwhelmed. First work with breath, because breath is the foundation. Use the hand-on-upper-abdomen technique, if needed, to help her establish a flowing breath pattern. Then observe her face.

If she is holding tension, choose one area of the face to work with. Choose the eye, forehead, jaw, or mouth. If you use a touch-and-say to help her relax her eye, then her jaw, then her forehead, all in one session, she will feel like you are ordering her around. She'll think you don't have a clue as to what she is dealing with and she will get perturbed with you.

If she relaxes one portion of the face, it affects the whole. You may only work with one area of the face during the entire labor. Your job is done when you point out tension with a touch-and-say. It is not your job to make her relax. Monitor your own breath and be there as the mountain. Come back to it later. Be sensitive to her capacities, and do not overwhelm her with something she cannot do in that moment.

You can also help your partner by monitoring facial tension *during* the contraction. For example, if her eye tenses, use a touch-and-say to help her relax. If she can relax her eye in the midst of her contraction, she will. If not, let it be until the wave is over, and help her relax between waves.

DO LABOR ONE WAVE AT A TIME

If your partner comes out of one rattle-your-teeth wave, and does not release the tension from it, she goes into her next one dragging the past with her. No one has the resources to do labor when they drag tension from the previous wave into the next, and then the next. Accumulating tension, rather than letting it go, is a prescription for being overtaken by the force of labor. This is why monitoring your partner's breath and facial tension both during and between contractions is crucial assistance.

After her wave is over, encourage her to take a cleansing breath and let the tension wash away with an exhalation or with sounding. Say to her: *That wave is over. Let it go.* Use hand-on-upper-abdomen technique to help her establish a fluid breath pattern. Choose one area of the face, and use a touch-and-say to help soften her face. If you assist the mother to release tension between contractions, she enters her next one with less tension.

These techniques help the mother to let go of one contraction and prepare for the next. Use them to help her soften and release *during* the contraction too. Realize the mother may be unaware of her restricted breath pattern and facial tension during labor, unless you point it out.

Most women are capable of doing labor one breath, one wave at a time. Women get overwhelmed when they do not release the last wave before the next and may need drugs to help them get through. Your assistance can be the crucial factor that allows your partner to navigate labor without pain medication.

HOT SPOTS

In the midst of labor, your partner will likely hit *hot spots* of accelerating labor. This is the scenario: your partner is in an intuitive space and is working well with labor. But suddenly labor accelerates; you notice because her breath pattern alters. Now she is either attempting to run in an effort to escape, or she is resisting by pitting her energies against its powerful, convening force. She is dragging her last wave with her instead of releasing it.

Labor is like stairsteps. There is an incline, then a plateau. Another challenging incline, and another plateau. The inclines get steeper and more intense as labor progresses. The plateaus get shorter. However, in deep labor, the incline can go straight up, off the charts, without a plateau. Sometimes women are very close to pushing when this happens and do not know it.

During an incline of accelerating labor, your partner tends to lose it. During these inclines, your partner may lose her perspective and begin to doubt her ability to *do* labor. If this happens, intervene. First, use hand-on-upper-abdomen technique to help get her breath flowing again. Reassure her. Try sounding technique to support her breath flow and use the facial touch-and-say. Help her change her position (more on that later). Or use the countdown described below.

FIVE-TO-ONE COUNTDOWN FOR ACCELERATING LABOR™

If your partner is in a hot spot of accelerating labor, use the *five-to-one countdown technique*™. Since labor is like stairsteps with inclines and plateaus that become increasingly more intense, you can use this method to help her get through a tough incline and onto the next plateau. To use the five-to-one countdown technique, get close to her and say: *Let's do five more waves and if it's not better, we'll do something else.*

If she is in a hot spot, she may feel like she is being overtaken by labor. She may think it is only going to get worse from this point, get discouraged, and request drugs. By giving your partner a number, you give her a finite frame of reference. Stephanie shared: *As soon as my husband told me five contractions, I thought, 'Five? I can do five. I just can't do forever and five.'* Five is a number she can work with.

When the first wave begins, say: *Here's wave five,* and start counting it down. *Ten, nine, eight. You're doing great! Seven, six, five. We're halfway through. Four, three. Almost there. Two, one. Great job! You did it! Now we only have four more to go.* Then, between the waves, help her connect to breath by using hand-on-upper-abdomen technique, and use a touch-and-say to help her relax.

If your partner is distracted by the countdown during the wave, be silent during the contraction. For example, say: *This is wave four.* Then be silent until the contraction is over. After the wave is over, say:

You did great. That wave is over. Let it go. Encourage her to take a sighing exhalation. Use a touch-and-say or hand-on-upper-abdomen to help her prepare for the next contraction. Continue the countdown between waves until you get to the last wave. On the last wave say: *Only one more to go.* You may need to use hand-on-upper-abdomen technique during the wave to keep her focused on the breath.

If she has not gained her confidence after the five-to-one countdown, encourage her to do five more and combine the countdown with sounding. Couples often do several rounds of five-to-one countdowns in a row. If she does not want to count waves, try a different position. Get her into water or into the bathroom. Keep in mind she may be closer to the pushing phase than anyone realizes.

The five-to-one countdown has been used successfully by many of my clients. It was forged in the heat of one particularly difficult labor, where my client had gotten so overwhelmed that nothing I did was able to draw out her participation. Catherine commented on how the five-to-one countdown worked for her: *I got to this point where I couldn't go on. I couldn't do it, and I was mad because I couldn't get out. But the countdown helped me stay with it.*

Men have an inherent understanding of encouraging their partners to continue through the countdown. Jeremy shared: *The five-to-one countdown was the only thing that worked for my partner once she started requesting drugs. We managed to get through without them, but I don't think we would have made it without drugs if we didn't have a technique that helped us. Once we finished one round, we started another, and it helped her focus and stay with it until the end.*

BREATHE-IN-BREATHE-OUT TECHNIQUE™: AT THE NOSE

Your partner may arrive at a point where labor is accelerating too rapidly for her to assimilate. She gets overwhelmed by the enormity of it and none of the tools work. Judith expressed how she felt overtaken by labor: *At one point, I felt like I was literally drowning in labor. There was nowhere that labor was not. I was being swallowed by labor. I didn't care what they did to me. Just knock me out. Just get me out of here. But I couldn't talk. Shortly after that, I started grunting and then I started to push and the whole thing immediately changed. I was so close and didn't know it.*

If nothing works, your partner may be very near the end. She may be in transition labor and making the last major incline. Soon she will be pushing, but no one may realize she is in transition. She may be shutting down her breath in an attempt to escape the drowning waves and the extreme intensity of labor. In those instances when she is beyond her edge, once you have gathered your composure, try *breathe-in-breathe-out technique*™.

Between contractions, touch the tip of her nose and say: *Focus on the tip of your nose.* Lean close to her and cue her by saying: *Breathe in. Breathe out. Good job.* Continue cueing her to breathe in, breathe out through the duration of the contraction. Don't be concerned with getting the breath to the diaphragm or any other technique. A jerky, grabbing breath is better than stopping the breath and shutting down. The main idea is to keep the breath moving in and out at the tip of the nose, so she does not stop breathing and drown.

Reassure her. Between the waves, if she has capacity to deepen her breath or soften her face, assist her. However, she may not be able to do it if her focal point is the tip of the nose and she feels like she is drowning in labor.

Not every woman experiences this intense response to her labor. Depending on the labor, you may not need to use the breathe-in-breathe-out technique at the nose. But if this is where your partner is, you need to meet her. This technique can be effective in assisting her through the last phase of labor.

CHAPTER 11

WHAT ARE FOCAL POINTS AND HOW DO I USE THEM?

A *focal point* is a point of reference that your partner can focus on to help her manage and cope with contractions. It keeps her connected to her body, helps center her attention during the contraction, keeps her from being overwhelmed, and reduces pain. A focal point may work through much of labor, or it may work for a while and then no longer work. When something ceases to work, it's useless. Discard it. Move onto a different technique. Focal points mentioned in the previous chapter are listed below:

1. Breath awareness, both during and between the waves of labor
2. Hand-on-upper-abdomen technique, with the focus on breathing into your hand
3. Sounding with the exhalation, focusing on the *aaahhhh* sound
4. Using a touch-and-say, focusing on the eye or jaw, to relax (This is a temporary focus.)
5. Five-to-one countdown
6. Breathe-in-breathe-out technique, at the tip of the nose—only when nothing else works

Below are other helpful focal points. These start with early labor and move through transition. Working with early labor waves gives your partner a map of how to work with the more challenging waves of active labor.

CERVIX-BREATHING™ FOR EARLY LABOR

Once early labor contractions begin to grab your partner's attention, help her into a comfortable supported position like a frog, a squat, a supported all-fours, or sitting on the ball. (*See* Chapter 16 for descriptions of these positions.) Then suggest she use the cervix as a focal point. She breathes through the nose on both the inhalation and the exhalation. As labor becomes more intense, she inhales through the nose and uses sounding with the exhalation. With the in-breath, she breathes into and through the cervix, visualizing opening. With the out-breath she breathes out of and through the cervix, visualizing opening while she consciously releases tension.

This *cervix-breathing technique*™ is excellent to use in early labor. It gets her breath working with labor, keeps her focused, connects her to her body, and calms the nervous system. In addition, it may relax and open the cervix. Cue her with words like: *Open. Give. Surrender.*

Your partner may use cervix-breathing with each wave, or she may use it intermittently. Let early labor be about expansion, opening, and release. Offer fluids. Take breaks when needed. Encourage her to change positions regularly.

COMBINE BREATHING WITH PELVIC ROCKING

Your partner can also combine breath with pelvic rocking. Use pelvic rocking in frog position, in all-fours positions, in a modified standing position, or on the ball.

Exhaling, she rocks the pelvis forward. Inhaling, she rocks the pelvis back. Combining the breath with gentle rocking movements of the pelvis focuses and stabilizes your partner in early labor and may relieve back pressure.

DIVE-INTO-PRESSURE TECHNIQUE™

Another focal point is the sensation of pressure. Instead of pulling away from pressure or pain, she dives right in. She uses her attention to actively breathe into the contraction. The inhalation penetrates through the gripping pressure, softening it. The exhalation releases and moves it out.

Some women use this technique throughout labor. When the *dive-into-pressure technique*™ works, it tremendously reduces pain. Instead of interpreting a contraction as pain, the mother is able to interpret it as pressure. She uses the inhalation to consciously penetrate the pressure. She uses the exhalation to consciously release pressure and move it out of her body. Some women are so effective with this technique the nurses are not convinced their patient is in active labor.

Here is Ann's story:

I went to the hospital in the middle of the night. When the nurse examined me, I was two centimeters dilated and she was convinced I was having false labor. But I was determined to have my baby. At my in-

*sistence, the nurse let me spend the night. I dove right into each wave,
softening with the inhalation and releasing with the exhalation. I was
managing the waves so well that in the morning the nurse thought I
was still in false labor, so she brought me breakfast. She told me after
I ate the doctor would examine me and send me home. But my doula
and I knew I was in active labor, so my husband ate the food. When the
doctor examined me, I was at seven centimeters, and the nurse had no
clue I was in real labor! The baby was born three hours later.*

Cue your partner to dive into the pressure as long as it works.
The dive-into-pressure technique allows your partner to use her attention to consciously and productively work with labor, and greatly
reduces pain.

DIAPHRAGM: GO TO THE BEACH

If the convening and converging forces get too powerful, your partner
will not be able to use either cervix-breathing or the dive-into-pressure as a focal point. You will know when to help her switch focal
points because her breath and behavior change. She gets agitated.
She may tell you to screw this cervix or dive-into-pressure idea because it doesn't work for real labor. When something ceases to work,
it's useless. Throw it out.

At this point, the waves are so strong that she is better off getting out of the way of the contraction. Labor has gotten so big that
her participation with the sensation in the pelvic region no longer
works. Her best strategy is to let body wisdom guide the work of the
contraction in the pelvic region and *go to the beach* in the diaphragm
region.

Remember how the rocks at the shoreline of the ocean are hit
with a much more powerful force than the sandy beach? The image is
to help your partner lie low—like lying in the sand at the beach. Cue
her by using hand-on-upper-abdomen technique and say: *Go to the
beach and lay low.* Her goal is to focus on her breath at the diaphragm,
lie low, and let the waves of labor wash over and through her with as
little resistance as possible. She gets out of the way of the contraction
in the pelvic region, centers her attention in the diaphragm region,
and gives labor free reign to do its work.

CHAPTER 11

USE A CHOSEN WORD OR PHRASE

Using a **chosen word or phrase** as a focal point is a shortcut in labor. Your partner needs to let you know if there is a word or phrase that is *weighted* for her. Some women have a habituated psychophysiological reaction to a specific word or phrase they have used over and over again in prayer, chanting, hymns, or meditation. Cueing your partner with a weighted word or phrase is like offering a guiding light to help find her way through a particularly challenging wave or period of labor.

When I was in labor, I used the word *rest*. When my husband said the word *rest*, I had a prewired response because I had practiced relaxation using that word repeatedly. It also reminded me to rest in God, so it made me feel safe.

If your partner has no chosen word, and most women do not, bend close to her ear and say: *Soften.* Most women have a psychophysiological response to the word *soften*. Their nervous systems respond to the word and assist them to relax and soften in the midst of a wave. Below are a few other phrases you can use during labor:

- *Lie in the sand at the beach and let the waves wash over and through.*
- *Go deep.*
- *Flow with the breath.*
- *Be still like a mountain and flow like a river.*—attributed to Lao Tse Tung
- Any other word or phrase you are instinctively drawn to use.

These phrases give your partner an idea of how to work with labor. She may want to repeat her word or phrase, like a ritual or a mantra.

If your partner has a connection to a personal God, remind her that God is present and attending her. Any idea that helps your partner stabilize or feel secure facilitates labor. She may want to repeat her Lord's name over and over again. Since birth is a life-altering, spiritual experience, it is natural that the Lord to whom she is connected be invited to attend her. If this idea has no strengthening appeal for her, you won't use it.

MOVEMENT RITUALS: PATTING, STROKING, OR ROCKING

Patting or stroking your partner's back, shoulder, forehead, inner thigh, or another place you are instinctively drawn to pat or stroke can soothe her. A firm, steady stroke is more stabilizing than a light stroke and lets your partner know you are solidly with her. However, some women cannot stand to be unnecessarily touched. Be sensitive to your partner's cues. Touch your partner from a calm space. Sometimes men pat from a place of nervous energy, and it is a fidgety pat that is distracting or jarring. If you see your touch is disturbing her, stop.

Patting, stroking, or rocking to soothe, like sounding, is universal and hardwired into us. Parents instinctively soothe a baby by patting the baby's back or rocking the baby. You may have an instinctual knowing of when and where to pat or stroke your partner. Move on that instinct if it arises. Some women get into a movement ritual during labor and want the same movement repeated time and again. One example of a movement ritual is rocking.

Cynthia shared how important the rocking ritual was to her: *What helped me most was rocking on the ball. I got into the shower and took the ball in with me. I sat under the shower and started doing this side-to-side rocking move with the contractions again and again while I groaned. I stayed in there a long time. My husband, when he realized I wasn't coming out, got his swimsuit on and joined me. He helped me rest between contractions by having me lean against him. Sometimes he pressed into my lower back. But when a contraction started, I needed to rock. Finally, the midwife came in and asked if I would come out so she could check me. I didn't want to leave, but I did. Not long after that, I was pushing.*

PRESSURE POINTS

Another technique is to press into pressure points during the contraction. One is the soft area between the base of the thumb and first finger. Use your thumb and first finger to press behind the webbed area into the muscle tissue between the base of her thumb and first finger. Helen shared: *At one point, all I wanted was for my partner to press as hard as could on the pressure point in my hand.*

Trevor, her partner, commented: *I thought I was going to pinch through her skin, but she kept saying, 'harder, harder.'*

Helen added: *For whatever reason, that was the additional stimulation that enabled me to get through that intense period of contractions.*

Another point is directly beneath the center of the ball of the foot. Press firmly into the point during the length of the contraction. Use other pressure points you are instinctively drawn to. If you have someone else with you, they can assist by pressing on pressure points. You can also use counterpressure on the lower back during contractions or pressure on her hip joints. (*see* **Figure 11.1**)

Some women find additional pressure focusing. Others find it distracting. Be sensitive to your partner's response.

ONE TOOL AT A TIME: TRUST YOUR INSTINCTS
The value of all these tools is they help the mother focus and stabilize. They also reduce pain. The most effective way to do labor is one breath, one wave at a time. All these strategies connect the mother to her body and assist her to stay in the present, in the now. In some cases, a single tool or technique may be effective through the entire labor. In other cases, a tool may work for a while and then have a diminishing effect. Discard what no longer works and use a different technique. Be practical. Adapt to the mother's needs. Trust your instincts.

USE DIFFERENT POSITIONS IN LABOR
Do not dismiss the value of helping your partner change positions regularly during labor. Chapter 16 includes a detailed list of positions commonly used in labor. Combine the intervention tools discussed in Chapters 10 and 11 with different positions.

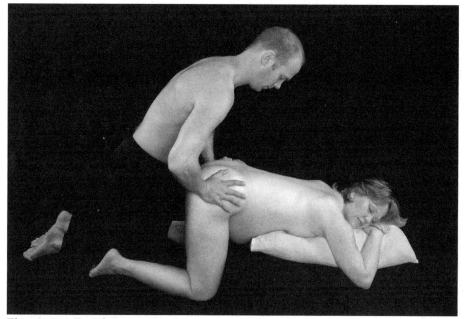

Figure 11.1 Besides pressing on pressure points during labor, you can also use counterpressure on your partner's hips, if it feels good to her.

CHAPTER 12
WARRIOR SKILLS TO PROTECT YOUR SPACE AND HERS

HANDGRIPPING: PROTECT YOUR SPACE

In the thick of labor, some women become serious handgrippers. If your partner tethers you in the infamous handgrip of labor, you will not be able to be a warrior and protect her space. This is why you need to know how to protect *your* space if she morphs into a handgripper.

Sally shared her need to hold on: *I grabbed onto my husband's shirt and couldn't let go. After the baby was born, my hands were sore, and his shirt had these two wrinkled, tight bulges that stood straight up by his shoulders.*

Nate, her husband, responded: *You were hanging on so tight I could barely move. You pulled me over, and I stayed there even though my back was killing me.*

Alexander shared his story of being caught in the grip: *My wife grabbed onto my first two fingers and hung on as tight as she could. I swear she twisted my fingers and tried to break them. It was the worst part of labor for me.*

His wife Nora commented: *Honey, you had no idea. It was so hard for me. I wanted you to know.*

Handgripping is a coping mechanism and a way for the mother to focus her attention and connect with her partner. However, it can morph into purposely squeezing or pulling as hard as she can to let her partner know how intense the pain is. This is one of the quirks of human nature; we want others to share our pain. Women are in a tremendous undertaking, and some want their partner (who got them pregnant, mind you) to know what it feels like for them.

A woman who practices relaxation regularly during pregnancy more effectively uses relaxation during labor. However, some women cannot relax their hands during labor; they need to hang on by tightly gripping. If your partner is wired to be a handgripper, give her handgrips and encourage her to hang on. Below are three ways you serve yourself and your partner by protecting your space, giving her handgrips, and not allowing yourself to be tethered or in pain:

- First, when you are tethered by the handgrip, you lose both your mountain and your warrior stance. You also lose your mobility and cannot respond to your partner in other mean-ingful ways.

- Second, the more comfortable you are, the more comfortable she is. If she is hurting you in the notorious handgrip of labor, it doesn't help either of you. When you are uncomfortable, it does not help the mother in any way.
- Third, securing her hands with grips gives her a much-need-ed something to hang onto and protects her hands from be-ing painfully sore after labor. It also prevents you from being tethered, uncomfortable, and otherwise useless.

Do not take this to an extreme. This does not mean you should not hold your partner's hand or allow her to grab you and hold on. Sometimes holding onto you is exactly what she needs. Holding onto one another may be the best way to stay connected and to transmit your strength and reassurance to your partner. It lets her know you are tangibly with her and makes her feel safe. The point is not to al-low yourself to get tethered and uncomfortable because that serves neither of you.

You know your partner and you know yourself. Go with it. But pack handgrips in your departure bag. If you get tethered, you will have them available.

WHAT ARE HANDGRIPS AND WHERE DO I GET THEM?
Make handgrips by using two six-inch rulers or cutting a paint stirrer into six-inch lengths. You will need two grips, four washcloths, and cloth tape—the kind gymnasts use. Take two washcloths, put them together, fold them in half, and wrap them tightly around the ruler. Then wrap the length of the grip securely with cloth tape. The grips you craft with the cloth tape are firm. They also stimulate acupressure points in your partner's hands, which may decrease pain levels.

You can also purchase handgrips. Training grips are sold in sports stores. Toy stores sell soft, squeezy stars and balls, which work as grips. Drugstores sell egg-shaped or oblong grips filled with sand or other materials. Remember to buy two; you will need one for each hand. You may choose to take a few varieties.

If you do not have handgrips and need them, take six washcloths, three for each hand. Fold them in half, roll them tightly, and give them to your partner to hold.

RUNNING-INTERFERENCE TECHNIQUE™: PROTECT HER SPACE

You spare your partner tremendous loss of energy, minimize distractions, and free her to concentrate exclusively on labor by using the *running-interference technique*™ and being a go-between for communication between your partner and the staff. Lucy shared: *A nurse came in to ask me a question. She stood at the end of the bed and I was wondering, 'Why is she talking to me from so far away? Doesn't she know I'm in labor?' I made this Herculean effort to come out of my labor enough to understand her. Then I could barely respond.*

In a scenario like this, your partner needs you to be her warrior and protect her space. During deep labor, your partner processes external information within a twelve-inch radius of her face. Beyond that radius, it takes much more effort for her to understand what is being said. You are in a position to communicate intimately with your partner, and she trusts and knows you, which adds to her sense of protection.

When the staff asks your partner a question, turn to the staff person and respond by saying: *Just a minute. I'll ask her and let you know.* If she is the middle of a contraction, wait until the contraction is over to ask. Get close to your partner and relay the information. Your partner responds to you; you minimize the work she has to do to deal with the intrusion. You can then turn to the staff person and relay information from your partner.

Occasionally, your partner is in a hot spot of labor and any request is more than she can handle. She may whimper: *I can't.* Or she may utter a decisive, edgy: *No.* She may snap: *Not now.* In that case, say to your partner: *We'll wait.*

That lets you respond to your partner's current need, and you turn to the staff person and say: *She needs a few minutes.* After a few contractions, your partner may hit a plateau and be able to respond to the staff's inquiry. If she does not hit a plateau after a few contractions, and they are there to check her dilation, announce to your partner you are going to help her get into position so they can check her. No need to ask again.

Be courteous to the staff. You do not want to alienate them, because they are there to help you if you need them. The staff and you are both interested in the same result: a healthy baby and a healthy mom. They are often busy doing their jobs and are not necessarily cued in to your partner. Being cued in to your partner is your job. Making critical comments to or copping an offensive attitude with staff does not help your partner. Keeping everything courteous and unruffled helps your partner maintain her confidence.

By using running-interference technique, you free your partner from unnecessary distractions, conserve her energy, protect her space, and make a valuable contribution to labor. Immanuel shared how rewarding it was for him to be able to protect his partner's space: *There were just a few times when my wife came out of labor to deal with the real world. Otherwise, she was inside where she needed to be. Being watchful, running interference, and protecting her space so she could stay inside was really important to me.*

LET THE STAFF KNOW YOU ARE RUNNING INTERFERENCE

If you use running-interference technique in a hospital birth, let the staff know you will be a go-between for communication. They may adjust their behavior to speak directly with you. However, do not assume the staff will remember this request. They will often address your partner, regardless.

Go ahead and run interference for your partner, and deal with the staff in a courteous manner. Assume they are busy and do not intend to disregard your request. Do not take it personally or be offended, but do not let the staff distract you from using the running-interference technique when your partner needs it.

HOW TO RUN INTERFERENCE ON PAIN-MEDICATION INQUIRIES

Hospital nurses enter the room specifically to inquire about pain medication. If you and your partner have the intention of using drugs only if necessary, then asking your partner if she wants drugs is like giving her an invitation to take them. If your partner is coping, even though it is challenging, deal directly with the staff without asking your partner.

Marie shared how her partner dealt with the staff during pain relief inquiries: *Without asking me, he kept telling the nurse, 'No thank you; she's doing okay.' If it weren't for my husband, I would have had drugs.*

When a woman needs pain medication, she generally asks for it without being prompted. If your partner has a desire to get through labor without drugs, your support is essential. In the heat of labor, without you running interference, your partner may opt to get out of the fire. I do not want to give the impression your partner should not use pain medication; it is a personal choice. But it is judicious to let your partner be the one to ask. Next is an entire chapter on how to be wise with drug choices.

CHAPTER 13
PAIN AND MEDICATION: MAKING WISE CHOICES

PAIN AND DRUGS:
YOUR SUPPORT CAN MAKE THE DIFFERENCE

Some women make the decision to use pain medication before the onset of labor. Others prefer to do labor without medication, but are open to using it, if needed. And some are committed to getting through labor without drugs. But the level of support a mother receives frequently influences whether drugs are used. You are often the one who makes the critical difference.

The medical staff on a labor wing of a hospital deals with birth every day. Their experience has taught them that many women who intend to go through labor without drugs request drugs once they are in the heat of labor. However, if you have a solid stance, abide in it, and demonstrate your skills by remaining grounded and focused; you impact how the staff responds to your partner's labor, as well as how your partner responds to pain.

In some labors, pain medication eases the mother through an exhausting or overwhelmingly painful labor. In other labors, pain medication creates problems requiring intervention that would not otherwise have been needed. In rare instances, emergencies occur that make intervention necessary. But if labor is progressing normally and your partner is coping, even at her edge, medication for pain can be detrimental.

It is possible the mother will make a drug request just as labor is rapidly advancing into transition, which is the shortest and most intense phase. Soon she will be pushing, but no one has a clue. It is the darkest hour before the dawn. Pain medication administered once your partner is in transition labor is problematic because it decreases sensation for pushing. It also increases the incidence of episiotomy, vacuum extraction or forceps, and cesarean birth. Many women experience the pushing phase as rewarding, and find a power and strength of which they were previously unaware. It is counterintuitive to have full sensation for labor, but then be numbed for the pushing phase.

TECHNIQUES TO USE TO ASSIST WITH PAIN

If the mother requests pain relief, you want to respond to her immediate need, but you also want to consider the larger picture. Confer with the staff to determine how dilated your partner is before administering pain medication. If you want to hold off on the use of drugs or if your partner expressed a desire to avoid medication, use the options below. Of course, if you are having a home birth, you will likely not have to deal with the decision of pain medication, but you can use these options to assist your partner to deal with pain. Use what you are instinctively drawn to use and discard the rest:

- Get her up to use the bathroom. Your partner must relax her pelvic floor to release her urine, and this may help get her through the impasse she is in.
- Monitor her breath. Is she using it to resist or run away from labor? Use the hand-on-upper-abdomen technique to help her focus and reestablish fluid breath flow.
- Monitor her face and use a touch-and-say to help her release tension.
- Encourage her to sound. Her sounds can be primal and roaring or subdued.
- Encourage a movement ritual like rocking on the ball; combine it with sounding.
- Use the five-to-one countdown technique several times in a row. She may be in a hot spot of accelerating labor and be able to cope again once she hits another plateau.
- Use touch, massage, acupressure points, or counterpressure on the lower back or hip joints.
- Use a chosen word or phrase.
- Change positions. Sometimes the baby is positioned in such a way that it creates additional pressure. When the mother changes positions, it encourages the baby to move, which may reduce pain.
- Get her into water. Encourage her to take a bath or a shower.
- Use cold or hot packs; you can also use them alternately.

The Gate theory of pain control explains why these strategies work to diminish pain. The theory is that perception of pain is altered or blocked by the brain when other stimuli are provided for the nervous system. By using a focus or other stimuli, the nervous system responds by blocking or lowering the perception of pain.

PAIN SERVES A PURPOSE IN LABOR

If you understand how pain serves the purpose of labor, it helps you remain calm as you try the pain relief options mentioned above. Henci Goer, in her book *Obstetrical Myths Versus Realities: A Guide to the Medical Literature*, reveals pain's purpose in labor: *Nerves in the cervix...pelvic floor muscles, and vagina, transmit stretching sensations as well as pain. These stretch receptors signal the pituitary to produce more oxytocin, which increases the tempo of the labor, causing further dilation.... Numb the nerves...and you wipe out the positive feedback mechanism.*[7]

Endorphin levels increase when your partner experiences pain. Pam England, author of *Birthing from Within: An Extraordinary Guide to Childbirth Preparation*, explains the potency of endorphins: *Endorphins are chemical compounds secreted by the brain and adrenal glands and have a pain-relieving effect ten times more potent than morphine.*[8]

Labor stimulates a dramatic increase of naturally occurring beta-endorphins, which is body wisdom's way of helping the mother to deal with and transcend pain. Endorphin levels in a birthing woman may increase by thirty times more than normal levels. Endorphins also help the mother get into an intuitive, altered state which helps her deal with labor.

Once pain medication is administered, the level of naturally occurring endorphins in the mother's system is reduced because the medication obstructs release of endorphins. When the drug wears off, pain takes on a greater intensity because of lowered endorphin levels. If your partner continues to labor without drugs, even though she is at her edge, body wisdom assists by producing higher levels of endorphins. It is also important to remain confident in your partner's capacity.

Deciding to use drugs is a judgment call. Sometimes the decision to intervene with drugs is the right one. Your goal is not to put off the drug decision indefinitely, but to try other alternatives first. If her drug request remains persistent, ask the staff to bring her something and support her 100 percent.

If she uses drugs, her mobility will be restricted. Get her up to use the bathroom before a drug is administered.

CHAPTER 13

REQUEST AN INTERNAL EXAM BEFORE ADMINISTERING DRUGS

If your partner needs pain medication, request an internal exam. Conferring with the staff can avoid administering a drug in the transition phase of labor. Mark's story illustrates the benefit of determining how dilated your partner is before administering drugs:

> We had a doula with us, but there came a point when my wife started demanding drugs. The staff brought in the stuff to do an epidural. But the doula encouraged me to ask the staff to do an internal exam. The staff said it wasn't necessary. Since they had just done an internal not long ago, they didn't want to do another one. But our doula continued to urge me to ask for an internal. At my insistence, the staff checked my wife, and she was at nine centimeters. When she heard she was nine centimeters, her whole demeanor changed. It was like this determination came out of her depths, and soon my wife was pushing. She pushed with such focus and power. I was glad I could do something that gave her the opportunity to have full sensation to push out our baby.

The hospital staff's primary concern is medical and life-saving support, and their role does not involve an intimate relationship with the unfolding waves of labor. The mother may be further along than the staff realizes. When a woman requests drugs, it is not always clear how close she is to the pushing phase. Requesting an internal exam can make the critical difference. It can determine whether your partner has full sensation during the pushing phase, and it can avoid unnecessary medical intervention and risk.

When you communicate with the staff, be straightforward but courteous, so the atmosphere around your partner remains free of unnecessary tension. Consider using the phrase that Denise Beaudoin, trainer of Portland doulas and former DONA trainer, recommends: *Is there a reason we can't try...?* This gives you the information you need, gives staff the means to move aside their habitual way of doing something, and gives you and your partner the information needed to do labor the way you both choose. For example, if your partner requests drugs, you can phrase your request: *Is there a reason we can't try checking her before administering drugs?* If they tell you it is unnecessary, inquire again: *I know it seems unnecessary, but is there a reason we can't do it?*

NARCOTICS, ANALGESICS, AND EPIDURALS

Narcotics and analgesics relieve pain during labor and are administered by a shot directly into the thigh or buttocks. They can also be administered through a vein via IV. The numbing effect lasts between two and six hours. They may make your partner sleepy, and she may experience a lapse of memory.

Epidurals are commonly used in hospital births. To administer an epidural, the anesthesiologist inserts a needle between the vertebrae of the lower lumbar spine into the epidura. The epidura lies next to the dura, which is the membrane that contains the spinal fluid and cord. The woman curves her spine to open space between the vertebrae. It is essential she remain still while the needle is being inserted, which can be difficult during a powerful contraction.

The anesthesia is sometimes administered as a single injection. Most commonly, it is set as a continuous drip through a catheter. It can also be self-administered through a push button. Your job is to ask for the push button. A woman who has an epidural needs both an IV and a fetal monitor. She is confined to bed, and will either need to use a bedpan or be catheterized to release urine. You can also inquire about a lesser dosage, which is designed to numb only the abdomen.

Some women decide before the onset of labor to have an epidural. Once the mother is four or five centimeters dilated, it is administered. She then has the benefit of pain relief through active labor. Other women decide to have an epidural after labor is under way and are greatly relieved once it is administered. If your partner chooses an epidural before the onset of labor, support her 100 percent. If you have used your skills during labor, and your partner decides she needs an epidural, support her 100 percent. For more detailed information on drugs and their effects, check out *The Birth Partner: Everything You Need to Know to Help a Woman Through Childbirth* by Penny Simkin, P.T.[9]

Epidurals can make a difficult labor manageable. Women generally recover from an epidural quickly and bond with their babies easily. Why doesn't everyone have one? It sounds like an epidural is the magic bullet of pain relief for labor. But there are some nagging concerns listed below:

- Confined to bed
- Tethered to an IV, a fetal monitor machine, and a spinal catheter
- Likely use of catheterization (inserting a tube into the bladder) to release urine before birth and possibly after birth
- May slow progress, requiring Pitocin to augment labor
- Diminished sensation to work with pushing contractions accompanied by less powerful pushing contractions, requiring a longer pushing phase
- Higher incidence of episiotomy
- Increased incidence of tearing of the perineal tissue
- Increased incidence of vacuum extraction or forceps
- Increased incidence of cesarean birth
- Increased incidence of infection requiring antibiotics
- Increased expense
- Experts are in control; loss of autonomy

When faced with an overwhelming labor or with an emergency that affects the health of the mother or baby, an epidural can be a Godsend. However, one downside to using pain medication is that a woman loses autonomy and an opportunity to uncover her internal power. A woman who has an epidural labors in a very different way than a woman who does not take pain medication. The contractions feel less intense and she does not have to be as engaged in her labor to manage pain.

Max compares and contrasts his partner's first birth with an epidural to the second birth without one: *In our first labor, my wife didn't have to cope with much pain because of the epidural. It was like we were just hanging around watching the fetal monitor and waiting for it to happen. But in the second birth we were both actively involved. It was a lot more challenging for us both. I had to stay focused, and we had to use a lot of skills. But she did great and it was more rewarding for us both because we felt like we did it. And we did it together.*

PITOCIN
If your partner's labor progresses slowly, stalls, or loses intensity, Pitocin may be used to stimulate or augment labor. Oxytocin is a natu-

rally produced hormone critical to beginning labor and sustaining contractions. Pitocin is a synthetic oxytocin that causes the uterus to contract. Pitocin makes the contractions more powerful and increases the intensity and pace of the contractions. In addition to Pitocin, your partner may need pain medication to help her cope with the increased intensity. That decision will be made based on how your partner manages.

Pitocin is also used to induce labor. If your partner or baby develops a medical condition toward the end of pregnancy, your medical caretaker may recommend inducing labor with Pitocin. For example, if your partner is leaking amniotic fluid, but labor does not begin within a reasonable length of time, your practitioner is likely to recommend induction. Once there is a tear in the amniotic sac, bacteria can get into the amniotic fluid, compromising the baby's and mother's health.

When Pitocin is used to induce, stimulate, or augment labor, it is administered through an IV. Monitors are necessary when Pitocin is administered to track contractions as well as the baby's heartbeat. The use of Pitocin is associated with an increase in medical intervention, as well as an increased risk of cesarean birth. Your medical professional will advise you and your partner if Pitocin is warranted.

If the staff recommends Pitocin during a stalled labor, but your partner wants to give labor a chance to progress on its own, ask the staff: *Is there a reason we can't wait before using medication?* If there is a risk, the staff will tell you, and you and your partner can make the decision based on knowledge. If there is not a medical reason, you give labor the opportunity to progress without intervention.

WHEN ARE DRUGS APPROPRIATE?

In the following scenarios, drugs are appropriate, but not always necessary, depending on the individual woman and her labor:

- A woman who chooses to use drugs from the outset and knows she wants whatever is medically available to help her.
- During a long labor, a woman may get exhausted and need pain relief to give her a reprieve so she can recharge before birth.
- Sometimes a woman fights labor with enough resistance that it is not progressing. Her pain escalates, and she becomes too frantic or discouraged to continue. In this scenario, drugs can

alleviate anxiety and help her relax enough for the cervix to open at a faster rate.

- During Pitocin-induced labors, pain medication can be helpful, depending on how the mother manages the contractions.
- The same is true for a stalled or nonproductive labor where Pitocin is used—again, depending on how the mother manages the increased intensity.
- A woman may hit the wall and not want to continue without pain relief.
- Pain medication will be used in a medical emergency that requires a cesarean section.

In all the above scenarios, pain medication can be helpful; it is an individual decision. However, if a woman is coping, even at her limit, pain medication may cause interventions that otherwise would not have been necessary. Keep in mind if your partner requests drugs, she may be closer to the pushing phase than anyone realizes. Women have an internal knowledge of what is best for them. Those choices may change as the situation unfolds. Your job is to be flexible, look at the larger picture, and support your partner in the choices she makes.

THE DRUG WITHIN
Birth presents an opportunity for a woman to discover her internal power. This unearthing of the forces within is the most powerful drug available. The great benefit of discovering her internal power is that for the rest of her life she knows it is available to her.

Melodie compared her first birth, in which she chose an epidural, to her second, unmedicated birth:

In my first birth, I went the epidural route at four centimeters, and it was a good birth. But in my second birth, I decided to see if I could manage labor on my own. In the middle of labor, I finally got that even though my husband and midwife were there for me, I was the only one who could pull this off, so I went deep. I didn't know the power that was in me until I dug deep. I realized that, while my first birth was wonderful, I sort of let others manage it for me. But in this birth I handled it on my own, and I discovered I could do it. It was a huge transformation in my psyche. Having dealt with labor, I felt like I could deal with whatever came up in the future.

Mae shared her method of diminishing pain in labor and discovering a deeper truth about her own being:

I practiced breathing and relaxation during pregnancy, and I was curious to know how it would affect labor. Once labor got under way, I focused on each wave and used my breath and sounding to release the pressure. I was able to interpret the waves as pressure, and I didn't think of it as pain. My focus went so deep that I submerged into an abiding part of my being. I realized it had always been with me, and I knew it would be with me forever. I don't think I could have uncovered that part of me if I hadn't been in a challenge that took everything I had to stay with it.

Bethany described benefiting from the challenge of labor:

I knew I wanted to do labor without drugs, and there was never a point where I felt like I needed them. I stayed focused by connecting to my breath. It was actually rewarding to face such a huge challenge and discover I could do it. I felt like I was being attended not only by my husband, but also by God, and I felt so much love. It sounds strange, but I never knew how much I was loved until I was in labor. After the baby was born, we were all enveloped in this grace and love. It stayed with us for weeks.

STORIES FROM WOMEN WHO CHOOSE MEDICATION

Below is Peter and Jane's story about their decision to use drugs during their first labor. I worked with them on their second labor, and they managed it without drugs. Jane told her story first:

I took classes with a birth educator who was totally against using drugs, and she went into all these details about how bad they were. I was influenced by her, and I was determined not to use drugs. But labor was so long and so globally painful that I couldn't relax, and I wasn't dilating. The pain kept mounting until I couldn't go on. As soon as the nurse gave me drugs, my body relaxed and I dilated at a faster rate. By

the time I was pushing, the drugs had worn off and I had good sensa-
tion and strength to push out my baby.

Her husband Peter presented his perspective:

When I saw my wife so reluctant to ask for drugs, I got angry at our
birth educator because my wife actually felt guilty about using drugs.
She was becoming exhausted and frantic. I told her I would help her do
whatever she wanted to do, and if she needed drugs, she should go for
it. The minute drugs entered her system, my wife started to relax. Drugs
helped her deal with labor. She was able to push the baby out without
any problems and they didn't need to use any medical interventions
during the delivery. The truth is, drugs didn't hurt the baby. And they
helped my wife.

Jessica shared her experience with deciding to use drugs deep
into labor:

I was determined to get through labor without drugs because I was con-
vinced it was the right way. But deep into intense labor, the staff did an
internal and told me I had a few hours yet to go. When I heard that, I
totally lost it and started demanding drugs. They may as well have said
your labor will continue forever. I knew I couldn't go on. I had made
my husband promise me he wouldn't let the staff give me drugs. But
at that point, I didn't care about anything I said. I just wanted out. We
were lucky, because by the time the nurse brought in the shot, I was
starting to push. That experience made me less judgmental, because I
realized no one knows what they will do until they are in the situation.

Marla shared her experience of making the decision to use pain
medication before labor began, and the satisfying results she experienced:

I knew from the minute I found out I was pregnant I wanted whatever
was medically available to help me with my labor. In my mind, it's the
only rational thing to do. I can't imagine why anyone would choose to
experience pain when medication can alleviate it. To me, people who
advocate no drugs for labor seem arrogant and intolerant. How can
they know what is right for someone else? But drugs definitely made

labor tolerable for me. By the time I checked into the hospital, my labor was already painful. Once they administered the epidural, I got immediate relief. By the time I was ready to push, I had sensation to work with my pushing contractions. The whole experience was great. I'd recommend an epidural to anyone who wants to minimize pain, and I'll do it with my next baby.

Serena shared her experience about making the decision to opt for pain medication:

I was open to using drugs if I needed them. I ended up hitting the wall and knew I wanted drugs—now! The drugs worked pretty fast. They definitely took the edge off. And I was able to cope again, so it felt right. But not long after that, they told me I was at ten centimeters, and the nurse wanted me to push, only I couldn't feel much. They gave me an episiotomy and had to use forceps to get the baby out. Everything turned out fine, and I was overjoyed when I saw my baby. But looking back, I realize that at the point I was demanding drugs, I had very little time to go and didn't know it. I wish I had known.

Every woman does whatever she needs to do to get through labor and deliver her baby. Any way a woman gives birth is cause to celebrate. New life is miraculous, no matter how it gets here.

WHAT IF A CESAREAN BIRTH IS NEEDED?

Women are designed to birth babies, and most women are capable of birthing vaginally. However, there are medical conditions and emergencies that necessitate *cesarean* births (surgical removal of the baby from the uterus). If the mother or baby develops a medical problem that puts either of them at risk, the medical practitioner may decide to schedule a cesarean birth to protect their health. In this instance, a couple has time to weigh the risks and prepare, which eliminates the urgency and psychic trauma of having emergency surgery.

If your partner needs a scheduled cesarean birth, you check into the hospital at the scheduled time. Your partner has blood drawn and is given a medical workup. You are given surgical clothing and a mask, but your partner will not need to wear a mask. You accompany her to the operating room, where she is prepped, given an epidural, and tented. You stand or sit (usually they provide a stool) close to your partner's head while the surgery is performed, and you can talk with one another.

The practitioner uses a scalpel to make a long horizontal incision along your partner's lower belly and uses clamps to hold the opening. You will be able to watch as they reach in and remove your baby from the womb. You can tell your partner how beautiful your baby is, and they will give the baby to you both as soon as possible, provided the baby's vital signs are good. You and your partner can hold the baby while your partner is stitched up.

When there is an emergency that requires a cesarean birth, neither of you have time to prepare. It is said that the shortest, but most harrowing journey is the journey down the birth canal. If your partner needs a cesarean birth to ensure her health or her baby's, it can be a Godsend. Even though the situation is urgent, in most instances you will be able to accompany your partner into the operating room. The staff will administer an IV and epidural in the operating room, unless your partner already has one. In dire circumstances, you may be left outside and if the mother does not already have an epidural, she will be given a general anesthetic.

A woman who has a cesarean birth needs more time to recover and more support after birth because she has to heal from major surgery. She may also experience doubt, sadness, or regret. Let her talk and share her feelings, which to you may sound crazy at times. Listen to her, and don't try to fix it.

CESAREAN STATISTICS AND HOW YOU CAN MAKE A DIFFERENCE
The National Center for Health Statistics reports that 29 percent of births in the United States are cesarean births. By comparison, only 5 percent of births were cesarean in 1970. How can it be that twenty-nine women out of a hundred now require a cesarean, when in 1970 only five out of a hundred required one? What caused the dramatic increase?

Part of the increase in cesarean births can be attributed to the risk of litigation. This is also one reason hospitals require IVs and electronic fetal monitors. If there is any concern something is going wrong, the doctor may feel compelled to pursue surgery. The better-safe-than-sorry adage applies more than ever to the health of the baby, thus the need to err on the side of caution. However, sometimes the information received from the fetal monitor is inaccurate and causes unnecessary intervention.

Insurance policy dictates much of the interaction between patient and doctor. Doctors and nurses are obliged to follow standardized procedures and are no longer as autonomous as they once were. Bureaucratic regulation, as well as the need for hospitals and doctors to reduce litigation and maximize profits, results in instituting policies that are not always in the patients' best interest. Every patient is a potential opponent should a lawsuit ensue. Because of that, the medical community must document *everything*. Doctors, midwives, nurses, and hospitals are overwhelmed by paperwork.

Although most women who have had a cesarean are capable of delivering vaginally on their next birth, some hospitals have policies that routinely prohibit or strongly discourage *VBACs* (vaginal births after a cesarean). Doctors practicing in these hospitals are under pressure to follow policy and may encourage their patients to have another cesarean birth.

It used to be that a woman with twins was allowed to deliver vaginally. Now that is rare. It has become standard procedure for women with multiple births to be given a cesarean. It also used to be that if a baby's position were breech (feet down, instead of head down), the obstetrician would attempt to deliver the baby. Now it is standard procedure to have a cesarean for a breech presentation. Why? One reason is because of the risk of litigation.

In addition, the high cost of obstetrical malpractice insurance has driven some obstetricians out of their practice and discouraged others from entering the field. Unfortunately, some hospitals have closed their labor and delivery wings because of the increased costs involved with both insurance and litigation. As a result, there are outlaying communities in the USA that no longer have convenient access to obstetricians or hospitals who can care for women during pregnancy and birth.

Surprisingly, another factor in the rising number of cesarean births could be the presence of the fathers, according to Michel Odent, MD, founder of London's Primal Health Research Centre. This does not mean fathers should not be in the labor room. However, it does mean fathers need to be mindful of the influence they have as they attend their partners. Odent explains: *When a woman gives birth, she needs to lose herself in the primitive or limbic part of her brain...The presence of an anxious father-to-be interferes with her mental state. By constantly asking "rational" questions, and asking his partner if she is all right, the man stimulates the intellectual part of her brain and interferes with the natural birthing process...In aiming to be protective of his wife, a man might suggest that she has an epidural or even a Cesarean so that she won't have too much pain.*

The concepts and practices in this book help you to relieve anxiety and give you tools you can use to provide support and refuge for your partner so you positively influence the outcome of birth. Your partner wants you with her, but she needs you to be her mountain and her warrior. You are in the rare position to offer her the protection and support she needs to have the best birth possible.

The bottom line is: there can be risks associated with the birth process. You and your partner's preparation provides the best approach toward taking advantage of what medicine has to offer without falling victim to unnecessary intervention.

PART THREE

PREPARATION PRACTICES

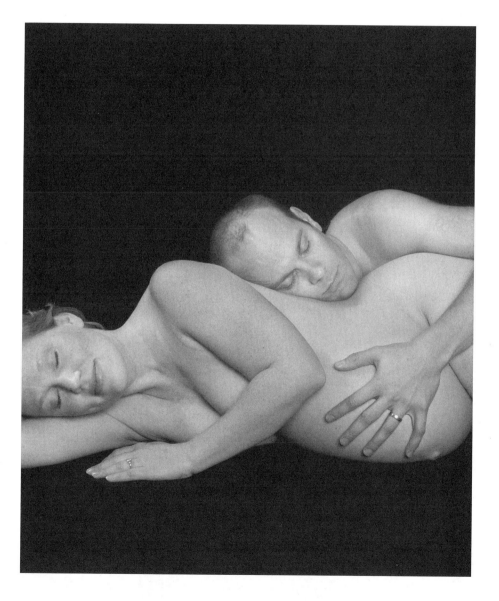

CHAPTER 14
BREATH, ALIGNMENT, AND RELAXATION PRACTICES

BREATH AND RELAXATION MAKE THE DIFFERENCE
This chapter provides breath and relaxation practices for you and your partner. Your goal is to practice breath awareness and become a fluid, diaphragmatic breather. If you both use diaphragmatic breathing, it will help you remain centered and reduce anxiety tremendously, as well as decrease pain for your partner. In addition, if you are aware of your breathing, you are more equipped to assist your partner with hers.

Included is a relaxation exercise. If you and your partner practice relaxation now, you will be more prepared to relax during labor. You will also have the opportunity to do a comparison between diaphragmatic breathing and chest breathing. Practice will help you detect if your partner switches to chest breathing during labor. You can then step in and use your skills to assist her. These simple techniques have the power to revolutionize how you and your partner experience labor.

PRACTICE DIAPHRAGMATIC BREATHING LYING DOWN
An easy way to observe your breath pattern is to practice while lying down. Practicing diaphragmatic breathing a few nights a week before you go to sleep is an easy way to become used to it. Your goal is to become a fluid and habitual diaphragmatic breather.

Your partner should also practice the breathing and relaxation exercises below, but because of the weight of the baby, she needs to lie on her side instead of her back to practice. Below are instructions to assist your partner in *side-lying position.*

ALIGNMENT IN SIDE-LYING POSITION
This is a position your partner may use during labor. To assist her alignment in side-lying position:
   1. Your partner lies on her side on a mat or carpeted floor. She can also use this position in bed to practice relaxation before

115

she goes to sleep at night. (The left side is traditionally recommended because the vena cava, the vein that returns blood from the lower body to the heart, lies to the right of the spine, and lying on the left side puts less pressure on it. However, she can lie on whichever side she prefers.)

2. Place a pillow under your partner's head so her spine is comfortably aligned with her head. If there are too many pillows under your partner's head, her head will be pitched at too high of an angle. If the pillow is too low, there is additional pressure on her neck and shoulder.

3. Then support the hip joints and legs by placing pillows between her legs and feet so that even the toes are supported. When you are in the birthing facility, if you cannot get extra pillows, roll up a few blankets. Place them between her knees and feet. Without support between the legs, there is additional pressure on the hip joints and lower back. By supporting her legs, feet, and toes, you reduce some of the work her body has to do to maintain its position, as well as help to relieve tension in the lower back and hip joints.

4. Once the length of her body is aligned and supported, wedge a rolled towel, blanket, or pillow into her lower back for support. Get her feedback on the back support and adjust it accordingly. Then offer a rolled blanket or pillow for her to hold onto to support the shoulder and arms. Does she need support anywhere else? Is she comfortable? Respond to her needs.

5. Again, observe her body from head to toe. The goal is to have a smooth, aligning flow from the crown of the head, through the tailbone, and down to the toes. But do not go for perfection. Go for comfort and support (*refer to* **Figure 15. 3**).

Once your partner is comfortable in side-lying position, you can both practice the breathing and relaxation practices below. Your partner adjusts the instructions as needed for her position. Here is the simple breathing practice:

1. Lie on your back on a mat or on a carpeted floor. You can also practice before you go to sleep, while you lie in bed. Either place a rolled towel at the base of the buttocks or place a pillow under your knees to relieve lower-back pressure. Place a thin pillow under your head.

2. Scan your body, align it to the best of your ability, and let it be comfortable.

3. Place one hand on the chest above the sternum. Place the other hand on the abdomen above the navel. (This is the space you will press into when you use the hand-on-upper-abdomen technique with your partner during labor).

4. Leave your hands in place and inquire: *How am I breathing?* Make no changes in the breath; simply observe how the breath moves. (*see* **Figure 14.1**)

5. Which hand rises and falls with the breath? If the hand on the chest rises, you are a chest breather. If the hand on your navel rises, you are a diaphragmatic breather.

6. If you are a chest breather, the goal is to establish a diaphragmatic breathing pattern. You can easily move breath to the diaphragm by stretching your arms overhead temporarily. This maneuver restricts chest muscle movement, allows the breath to move the diaphragm, and allows freer movement of the diaphragm.

7. After establishing movement of the breath at the diaphragm, press your hand into the area above the navel and breathe to your hand. Inhalation: hand rises. Exhalation: hand falls. The lower ribs flare slightly with the inhalation and retract with the exhalation. The hand on the chest remains still. This is diaphragmatic breathing, your goal.

8. Once you have established breath at the diaphragm, observe the quality of the breath. Is it jerky? Are there pauses? Are there noises? Focus on letting the breath flow freely without restrictions.

9. Gradually eliminate choppiness, noises, and breaks. Let it flow smoothly and rhythmically. Your goal is to become a fluid, smooth, diaphragmatic breather.

Practice as little as two minutes, or practice as long as you desire. Practicing before sleep sets your nervous system to continue breathing fluidly and diaphragmatically as you drift off. This helps you sleep better. It also helps you to learn diaphragmatic breathing at a faster rate with less work. If you practice breathing for one minute before you get out of bed in the morning, you start and end your day breathing diaphragmatically. This will help you learn more quickly. In a short time, you will be a fluid, diaphragmatic breather.

SIMPLE RELAXTION PRACTICE

After you have practiced diaphragmatic breathing, practice relaxation. Stay in the same position; your partner remains on her side and adjusts the instructions accordingly (She does not do numbers two and three in the following sequence). You can also practice relaxation before sleep. This practice starts with the head, moves through the body to the toes, and then moves back through the body from the toes to the head. Here is the simple relaxation practice:

1. Scan your body, align it to the best of your ability, and allow it to become comfortable.
2. Extend your arms, draw your shoulders away from your neck, and roll your head from side to side, releasing the shoulders and neck.
3. Your hands rest palms up, several inches away from your body and your legs and feet are separated. This is basic *sponge position* also called *shivasana*. (*see* **Figure 14.2**)
4. Close your eyes and let your mind occupy the space your body occupies. Release tension with an exhalation. Readjust so you are aligned and comfortable.
5. Allow the breath to flow diaphragmatically and focus on the smooth rhythm of the breath.
6. Bring your attention to the eyes. Let the eyelids gently close, and release tension in the tiny muscles that surround the eyes.
7. Release the corners of the mouth; release the jaw.
8. Soften and release the entire face.
9. Release the pit of the throat.
10. Release the shoulders, elbows, hands, and fingertips.
11. Release the fingertips, hands, lower arms, upper arms, and shoulders.
12. Again, release the pit of the throat.
13. Release the heart center and chest.
14. Release the navel center and abdomen.
15. Release the pelvic region and pubic bone.
16. Release the hip joints, knees, ankles, arches of the feet, and tips of the toes.

17. After reaching the toes, move back through the body. Release the tips of the toes, arches of the feet, calves, thighs, buttocks, lower back, upper back, the back of the neck, and crown of the head.
18. Let your whole body rest.

This relaxation practice can be done in as little as five minutes, or you can take a longer time and focus deeper. Relaxing before sleep helps you sleep more peacefully.

Go to the fathersatbirth.com web site and download a free twelve-minute guided relaxation practice. There is also a thirteen-minute pregnancy relaxation practice for your partner to download.

DIAPHRAGMATIC BREATHING IN SITTING POSITION

Both of you can experiment with diaphragmatic breathing in a sitting position:

1. Sit on the edge of a chair with your knees hips'-width apart and your feet flat on the floor.
2. Like a snowman, stack the three body weights—pelvis, chest, and head. Let your position be comfortable and aligned.
3. Lift your shoulders, roll them back, align them over the hips joints, and let them rest.
4. Pull a few hairs from the crown of your head toward the ceiling or imagine a string is pulling you from the crown toward the ceiling. This move adjusts and aligns the neck and head, and helps the spine align. When the spine is aligned, there is space between the vertebrae. The energy from the nervous system flows freely along the graceful *S* curve of the spine because the spine is not collapsed upon itself.
5. Place one hand above your sternum and the other hand above your navel. Observe the breath. Feel which hand rises and falls with the breath. If the hand on your chest is moving, raise both arms above the head temporarily. This maneuver unrestricts the diaphragm and allows it to move more freely with breath.
6. Press your hand into the area immediately above your navel. Breathe into your hand so that the hand moves out with the inhalation and in toward the core with the exhalation. The ab-

domen moves fluidly with the breath, but is neither rigid nor slack.

7. Once you establish breath at the diaphragm, allow the breath to become fluid, flowing, and unrestricted. With the inhalation the lower ribs slightly flare out and the belly rises, but the upper chest remains still. With the exhalation the belly moves in toward the core, the lower ribs slightly retract, but there is no movement in the upper chest.

8. Eliminate any exaggerated breaks or pauses and allow the breath to become smooth, flowing, quiet, and refined. Let breath be your only focus and let all else drop away.

9. Observe the calming, soothing effect diaphragmatic breathing has on the body and the focusing effect it has on the mind. You may discover that your alertness and sense of well-being increase.

This is an exercise, and you do not have to do it perfectly. If you try this experiment, you will both understand how diaphragmatic breathing reduces anxiety. If you experience it in your own body, you will be able to detect whether your partner is using diaphragmatic breathing during labor.

CHEST BREATHING
Now, experiment with chest breathing.

1. Remain sitting in the chair in the same position: one hand on the chest above the sternum and the other hand above your navel.

2. Take a series of shallow, jerky, chest breaths that cause the hand on the chest to rise and fall.

3. Keep the breath shallow and keep the belly tight.

4. Observe the anxious quality chest breathing produces in the mind and the tension it creates in the body.

5. Now hold your breath. Observe the effect of shutting down the breath. It lets you momentarily escape distress, but the result is increased anxiety and tension. (*see* **Figure 14.3**)

6. Continue using the chest to breathe in a shallow, jerky, noisy, restricted manner, and again hold the breath. If you continue in this breath pattern, you will discover over the course of a few minutes, distress and anxiety soar.

Chest breathing is not a good practice, so don't repeat this. The reason to do it is to compare it with diaphragmatic breathing. If you do chest breathing once, you both understand how chest breathing increases anxiety and pain for your partner during labor. If you experience it in your own body, it will be easier for you to detect if your partner uses chest breathing during labor. You can then step in and help her recoup a more productive breath-flow by using the skills in Chapter 10.

EXPERIMENT WITH MISALIGNMENT AND BREATH
Now experiment with how misalignment affects breath:
1. Sit farther back on the chair and slump over.
2. Observe the body and the breath. When the chest is collapsed, fluid diaphragmatic breathing is not possible. (*see* **Figure 14.4**)

The chest's collapse restricts breath, creates tension in the neck, and restricts optimal functioning of the internal organs and nervous system. Internal attitude alters; attention levels and even confidence diminish. Alignment affects you on many levels. If you practice, you will understand how comfortable alignment assists both of you during labor.

PRACTICE BREATH AWARENESS
To practice breath awareness, simply do the three-step, one-minute centering practice. Since breathing is a constant action, you do it on the spot, whenever you think of it. In short, you align and relax the body, let the breath flow diaphragmatically, and focus the mind.

Breath has the compassion and the wisdom to calm the body and focus the mind. If you become aware of your own breathing, and become a more fluid breather, it will help both of you during labor. When you are unsure of what to do or how to help in labor, tap into your breath (dive into your breathing), which is literally right under your nose whenever you need it.

Do not underestimate the power of the breath to assist you. Practicing breath awareness doesn't cost money. It doesn't take an act of faith. It doesn't take a degree. It takes a little instruction, a desire to do it, a little practice, a little perseverance—and that's it.

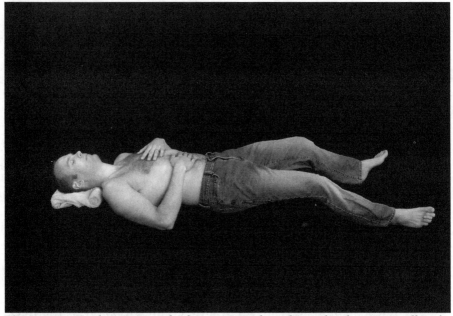

Figure 14.1 To determine whether you are breathing diaphragmatically, observe which hand moves when you breathe.

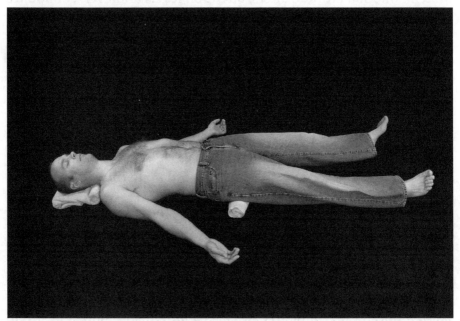

Figure 14.2 Shivasana, also called sponge position, is the basic relaxation pose, which you can do in bed or on the floor.

122

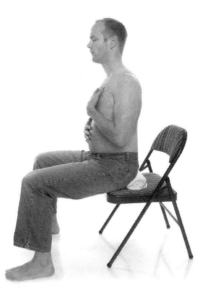

Figure 14.3 Align and relax the body. Place one hand slightly above the sternum and the other hand above the navel. Observe the breath and practice diaphragmatic breathing.

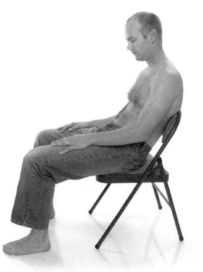

Figure 14.4 Observe how misalignment restricts your breathing, and has a detrimental impact on your entire system.

123

CHAPTER 15
SIMULATED HANDS-ON PREPARATION

This chapter presents hands-on simulated labor preparation exercises for you to do together. If you practice once together, it will influence how you both navigate through labor. Muscles have memory. If you do these once, your muscles will remember how to do them, and it will assist you both during labor.

SIMULATED-LABOR PRACTICE: WITHOUT FOCUS
This simulation practice gives you an opportunity to experience how focus alters your perception of pain. It also gives you an opportunity to experience how touch and talk either distract or enhance focus. Do this experiment twice, once without focus, once with focus, and compare the results. Then switch roles with your partner.

1. Begin by lying flat on your back on a mat or carpeted floor. Your partner sits next to you.
2. A pressure point lies directly underneath the ridge of the eyebrow bone. Use your thumb to press along the lower ridge of the bone until you feel a tiny indentation in the bone. The slight indentation is approximately three-eighths of an inch from the lower edge of the inner eyebrow. When you locate the point, you will know it because it is sensitive to pressure.
3. Have your partner press on the point as hard as she can. Most men discover that pressure on the brow bone point is uncomfortable. Many men get agitated or fidgety in an effort to escape. (*see* **Figure 15.1**)
4. While you are dealing with the discomfort, your partner continues to press hard while she talks to you, saying things like: *How are you doing? Is there anything you want me to do? You are supposed to relax your eye because if you relax your eye it will help you. Don't forget to relax your jaw. And don't forget to breathe, because that's important too. Is there anything else you need me to do?*
5. While talking, your partner touches and pats you with light, rapid, fidgety strokes on the forehead, face, and chest. (*see* **Figure 15.2**)

CHAPTER 15

This simulation gives men a mini-example of how much concentration and focus labor requires. It also gives them an idea of how fidgety touch and well-meaning, but unhelpful questions and instructions can get in the way. Joel said: *I was sort of dealing with the pain, but when she started talking to me and touching me, it made it worse.*

Alexander commented: *Whoa! And that was nothing compared to what my wife is going to go through!*

SIMULATION-LABOR PRACTICE WITH FOCUS: COMPARE THE RESULTS

Now try the simulation again using relaxation, focus, and breath:

1. Place a pillow under your knees to support your lower back and place a small pillow under you head. Lie in sponge position and get your body comfortable.
2. Place your hand above your navel and breathe into your hand until you establish a connection with breath. Inhalation: hand rises. Exhalation: hand falls. Allow the breath to become diaphragmatic, rhythmic, and flowing. Scan your body and release tension. Let it drop into the floor. Take a few minutes to practice the Simple Relaxation Practice from the previous chapter. While you relax your body and connect to breath, your partner focuses on her breathing and relaxes her body in any position she finds comfortable.
3. After relaxing and connecting to your breath, have your partner press on the pressure point in the eyebrow bone. Your partner presses firmly on the point while she observes you and connects to your breath.
4. She continues to press while she touches and talks to you, except this time the words and touch are direct and focused. She uses a solid, firm touch with hand-on-upper-abdomen technique as she says: *Breathe here.* She uses a touch-and-say to help you relax your eye.
5. Take your awareness to the point of pressure at the brow bone and use a diaphragmatic, fluid, flowing breath to breathe into and out of the point, dissipating the pressure.

Now compare results with the first simulation. Most men find that pressure and pain decrease. Some men remain so relaxed and focused that their whole awareness is the breath and they dissipate any experience of pain. Men make comments like: *I can't believe it. Are you sure you were pressing as hard?* Men comment that they could not believe the difference breath and relaxation made in coping with the pain, and make comments like: *I get it now.*

If you try this simulated-labor practice before birth, you get first-hand knowledge of how breath, relaxation, and focus make pain more manageable. It also gives you firsthand knowledge of how the power of touch and talk can either support or undermine your partner's focus.

TRADE PLACES

Now switch roles with your partner. The goal is for you to practice how to observe your partner's breath and how to touch and talk to her during labor. Practicing gives your partner the opportunity to tell you what she likes and dislikes. It also gives you an opportunity to learn how touch and talk support your partner's focus. Your partner needs to lie in side-lying position (*see* Chapter 14 for Alignment in Side-lying Position).

PRACTICE THE SIMULATION WITH YOUR PARTNER

Once you have helped your partner get comfortable in side-lying position, practice simulated labor with your partner.

1. You can either sit next to her on the floor, or remove the back support and use your weight to lean into and support her back. Do not use your body to support her at the expense of your own comfort. Make sure you are supported and comfortable. Use pillows to support your alignment. (*see* **Figure 15.3**)

2. Find the pressure point in your partner's eyebrow bone and press hard. Observe your partner's breathing. Experiment with soft gazing to witness the rhythm of your partner's breath while you press. Breathe with her so you know her breath rhythm in your own body. Observe the tension levels in her face.

3. Stop pressing and get her feedback. Tell her what you observed in her behavior and let her share how it felt in her body.

4. After exchanging feedback, give her a moment to scan her body, adjust her position, get comfortable, and release any residual tension.

5. Use the hand-on-upper-abdomen technique and ask her to breathe into your hand. Let her make any adjustments in your hand so it feels right to her. Encourage her to allow the breath to become fluid, flowing, and diaphragmatic. If she needs aid in moving the breath to her diaphragm, she can temporarily raise her arms above her head. (*see* **Figure 15.4**)

6. Encourage her to relax her face, which helps her whole body to relax.

7. Next, press hard on the brow point again. Encourage her to take her awareness into the pressure point and breathe into the pressure to dissipate the sensation of pain. Observe her breath and use the hand-on-upper-abdomen technique to assist her breath to stay smooth and diaphragmatic.

8. Observe any tightness in her eye and jaw. Continue pressing on the point while you use a touch-and-say to help her release tension in her face. For example, if her eye tenses, stroke the bone next to the eye, simultaneously saying: *Relax your eye.* Observe her reaction.

9. Release the pressure on the brow point. Encourage her to release any remaining tension with an exhalation like she is letting go of a wave of labor. Encourage her to soften her body and focus her mind on her breathing for a few moments.

10. Get her feedback and share your observations. Let her make any additional comments or requests.

If you practice this simulated labor, it gives you an opportunity to practice some of the skills you will use with your partner during labor; it also gives your partner an opportunity to experience how focus and breath can relieve pain during labor. In addition, your partner's feedback will give you a clearer understanding of how she needs you to touch and talk to help her maintain focus and minimize pain.

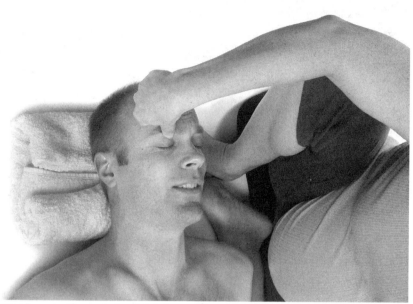

Figure 15.1 Locate the point, which is sensitive to pressure, on the lower ridge of your inner eyebrow and have your partner press on it hard.

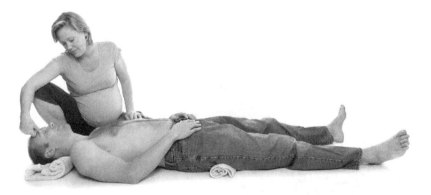

Figure 15.2 Have your partner continue to press hard on the eyebrow pressure point while she distracts you with questions, reminders, and unfocused touch.

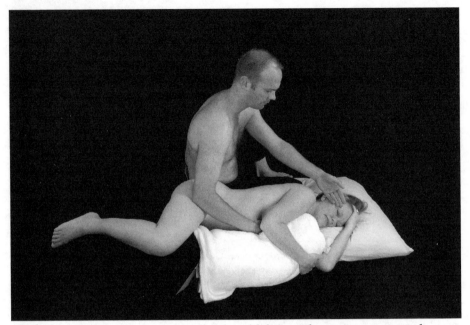

Figure 15.3 When you practice simulated labor with your partner, make sure you are comfortable, supported, and relaxed, because it helps your partner to focus.

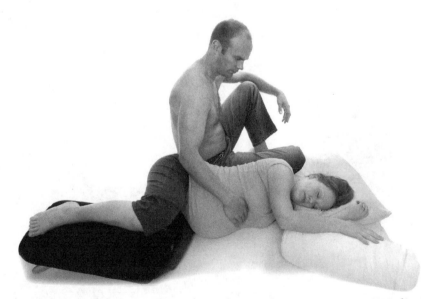

Figure 15.4 Use hand-on-upper-abdomen technique to encourage diaphragmatic breathing. Try breathing with your partner so you know the rhythm of her breath in your own body.

130

CHAPTER 16
LABOR AND BIRTH POSITIONS

POSITIONS FOR LABOR

This chapter provides labor and birth positions. There are a multitude of positions to use in labor, and like the focusing and breathing techniques you have practiced, each has benefits. However, a position may work well for a while, but then cease to be useful. A little advance homework to familiarize yourself with different positions can help you help your partner change positions when needed during labor. Practice positions at least one time together, and you will have more confidence during labor. During labor, you won't use all the positions; you may use only a few. Use what works and discard the rest. Below are positions with alignment details.

BASIC ALIGNMENT IN CHAIR POSITION

Most birthing rooms are equipped with rocking chairs, and your partner may do some of her labor in one. At home, your partner sits in any chair she chooses.

Once she is seated in *chair position*, observe her alignment. If the chair does not support proper alignment of the spine, her torso will collapse as she leans back into the chair. Besides causing neck strain, a collapsed torso restricts breathing and reduces abdominal space, putting additional pressure on her pregnant uterus. Place a pillow, blanket, or rolled towel behind her back to avoid collapse of the chest and torso. Observe her head. The head weighs twelve to fifteen pounds, and may need additional support. If the back of the chair is high enough, roll a towel and place it behind the mother's head or neck.

Observe her feet. Do they comfortably reach the floor? If not, there is additional tension in her lower back. To alleviate unnecessary strain in her lower back, support her legs by placing pillows or folded blankets on the floor for her to rest her feet on. Some birthing rooms have step stools you can place under her feet.

SQUAT POSITION WITH BREATHING

Squat position is highly recommended for pregnancy and birth. Some women are comfortable in a free-standing squat, but others need support. If your partner is not comfortable in a free-standing squat, find a wall space and put a few pillows on the floor next to the wall. Your partner sits on the pillows while she squats and uses the wall for support. Help her make any adjustments. She may need an additional pillow behind her back for support. (*see* **Figure 16.1**)

Once she is comfortable in squat position, encourage her to establish a smooth, rhythmic breath without pauses, noises, or jerks. Breathe with her. After establishing a flowing breath pattern, encourage her to squeeze, tighten, and contract her pelvic floor with the exhalation (like she is holding her urine). With the inhalation, she slowly releases and relaxes the pelvic floor. She is now doing deep rhythmic Kegel exercises for her pelvic floor muscles, in sync with her breathing. Use a touch-and-say to help her relax facial muscles. (Squat position, combined with breathing and tension and release of the pelvic floor muscles, is a valuable position to use during stalled labor.)

Once your partner has united the breath with the tension and release of the pelvic floor, she becomes calm and focused. Being calm and focused is extremely valuable in labor. Minimize distractions and avoid unnecessary conversation.

She can use squatting with the breath during early labor to focus her attention. (Once labor is active and advancing, she will no longer tense and release the pelvic floors.) Squatting during labor may help the baby move into a more optimal position, may encourage labor to progress if it stalls, and is an excellent birth position.

CAUTION

While squatting is highly recommended for pregnancy, labor, and birth, some women are not comfortable in a squat position. Some women have knee injuries, and for some squatting creates an uncomfortable level of pressure. If your partner gets into a squat and becomes uncomfortable or nauseated, help her get out of the position immediately. The most valuable positions are those in which your partner feels comfortable.

REVIEW OF BREATHING FOR SQUAT POSITION

1. Exhale—squeeze, tighten, and continue contracting the pelvic floor for the duration of the exhalation.
2. Inhale—slowly release and soften the pelvic floor.
3. The breath becomes rhythmic, fluid, and flowing without breaks, jerks, or pauses, which stabilizes the nervous system, calms the body, and focuses the mind.
4. Cue her to soften and release the face with a touch-and-say. Breathe with her.

BASIC ALIGNMENT ON THE BALL

If you have a ball at home, like those used in fitness programs, try the basic *ball position*. Stabilize the ball as your partner sits on it. Once she is seated, her legs need to be wide open to accommodate her belly, and her feet need to be flat on the floor for stability. Suggest she drop her tailbone to the earth, like an anchor, to ground herself. Then encourage her to roll her shoulders back, drop them, and center them over the pelvis for support. She can then pull a few hairs from the crown of head to lift and align the head. This aligns the spine and prevents collapse, so she can breathe effectively. The goal is for her to feel both grounded and lifted while sitting on the ball.

She can bounce a few times. During labor, this may encourage the baby to move down. Suggest she combine the ball with pelvic rocking—side to side, back and forth, or circling. Many women like to rock and circle the hips during pregnancy, as well as during labor.

Encourage your partner to combine pelvic tilting with the breath. On the exhalation, she rounds the spine, tilts the pelvis forward, and contracts (squeezes) the pelvic floor muscles. On the inhalation, she tilts her pelvis back and releases (relaxes) the pelvic floor muscles. (Once labor is active she may choose to use pelvic tilting on the ball, but she will no longer combine it with tension and release of the pelvic floor muscles.)

She uses the same basic breathing technique listed above under Review of Breathing for Squat Position above, except on the ball she is combining it with a pelvic tilt.

SUPPORTED ALL-FOURS POSITION

A *supported all-fours position* is a wonderful position for labor. All-fours positions take the weight of the baby off the spine and help relieve back pressure. Stack several pillows on the floor for your partner to rest her torso on. Assist her to get comfortable. Suggest she focus on her breathing and combine it with pelvic tilting.

This is also an excellent position for you to provide counterpressure or massage for her lower back. Get behind her and lean your weight into her lower back. While most women find lower back pressure soothing, some women do not. Joyce shared: *In my first labor counterpressure on my back felt so good, but in my second labor, my lower back felt like it was on fire and I couldn't stand for anyone to touch it.* (see **Figure 16.2**)

LIST OF LABOR POSITIONS

Below is a list of commonly used labor positions. While your partner practices these positions, observe her alignment and breath. You can also practice some of the intervention and focus skills described in Chapters 10 and 11 while you practice positions.

- **Walking**—Uses gravity and is an excellent position. During early labor, you can stroll with your partner outside, if weather permits. You can also walk through the birthing facility or your home once labor is under way.
- **Slow dancing**—Face one another; put your arms around each other like you are dancing and lean into one another. Sway back and forth.
- **Standing positions**—Your partner can do a simple standing position. She can also stand, place her hands above her knees, and lean into her arms for support. In this position, it is easy for your partner to combine standing with pelvic titling. Your partner can also do a standing pelvic tilt by placing her hands on the countertop. She uses it for support while she stands and rocks the pelvis, tilting it forward and back. Encourage her to combine the movements with her breath. (*see* **Figure 16.3**)
- **Supported back-stretch**—Your partner places her hands on a support like the kitchen counter, bends at the hip joints, and stretches her back. She can combine this position with pelvic rocking. You can also massage or provide counterpressure for her lower back in this position. This is a good position to relieve back discomfort. (*see* **Figure 16.4**)

- Rocking in a rocking chair—Most birthing rooms are equipped with rocking chairs. Make sure the chair supports her alignment. (*See detailed information in* **BASIC ALIGNMENT IN CHAIR POSITION**, *page 127.*)
- Sitting on a ball—Combine it with light bouncing, pelvic tilting, side-to-side rocking, or pelvic circling. (*See detailed information under* **BASIC ALIGNMENT ON THE BALL**, *page 129.*)
- Tailor sitting—Place a wedge or a pillow under your partner's pelvis to help keep the pelvis aligned and make her more comfortable. You can also stand behind her as she uses your body for support in tailor sitting.
- Squatting and supported squat positions—Your partner can do a free-standing squat, a supported squat against the wall, or she can hold your hands while she squats (lean away from her using your weight for support). Squat positions are excellent birth positions because they use gravity to move the baby out and encourage maximum opening in the pelvic outlet.
- Frog position—This is an excellent position for pregnancy and labor. She bends her knees so her legs are underneath her and opens her legs wide while she places her hands on the floor. This is an excellent position for pelvic rocking. You can also press your hands into her low back with your weight. (*see* **Figures 16.5 & 16.6**)
- All-fours and supported all-fours positions—All-fours positions are excellent for pregnancy and labor. In a traditional all-fours position, your partner gets on her hands and knees. She can tilt her pelvis and arch her spine like a cat. In a supported all-fours position, you stack pillows on the floor for her to rest her torso on. These positions help relieve back pressure and may help the baby move into a more optimal position, especially if the baby is in posterior position. (*see* **Figures 16.7 & 16.8.**)
- Side-lying position—Use for rest or deep labor. (*See* Chapter 14 for **ALIGNMENT IN SIDE-LYING POSITION.**)
- Be creative—This is by no means a complete list of positions. Feel free to experiment.

CHAPTER 16

HOW PRACTICE MAKES THE DIFFERENCE

Nathaniel commented how practicing the positions before labor gave him the confidence he needed to suggest changing positions regularly during labor: *Going through the practices and positions with my partner before labor really helped because I felt like I had a repertoire I could use during the different stages of labor.*

His partner Lindsey commented: *Once we were in the hospital, I started out lying on my side. I don't know that I would have changed positions if Nathaniel hadn't suggested it and helped me do it. That somatic experience of doing it in the body before labor is way different than having it in the mind. There is no mind in labor for the woman. I was out of my mind. So knowing it in the body is important.*

OPPOSITION MAXIMIZES OPENING IN PUSHING POSITIONS: PUSH-PULL TECHNIQUE™

The most common birthing positions are the semi-sitting and the squat positions. It is wise to practice these positions before birth. Opposition creates opening. By using opposition in the *push-pull technique* ™, your partner's pelvic outlet widens to allow the maximum space to birth the baby and gives her more control of the pelvic floor muscles during the pushing phase of labor.

PRACTICE SEMI-SITTING POSITION WITH OPPOSITION

Practice the semi-sitting push-pull technique together.

CAUTION: This position is safe and recommended for your partner to practice during pregnancy; however, she should not push (like she will when she is in pushing out her baby). She needs to avoid pushing in all the pushing positions you practice together below.

To practice the semi-sitting push-pull technique at home:

1. Sit on a mat or a rug and face one another.
2. Bend the knees and open the legs wide.
3. Place the balls of the bottoms of your feet against one another's. Heels are on the floor. (*see* **Figure 16.9**)
4. Contract the pelvic floor (the same muscle action you make when you hold your urine.) This is a basic Kegel exercise for the pelvic floor. It is not used during the actual pushing phase of labor, but it prevents your partner from pushing while practicing this position.

5. You both place your hands behind the knees and pull, while you simultaneously round the spine to create a **pelvic tilt** and push into one another through the feet. Pushing into one another with the feet while you pull with the arms creates opposition. Opposition creates a wider opening in the pelvis and gives the mother more space to birth her baby.

6. Keep the breath flowing.

By using the opposition of arms to pull and the feet to push against one another, you will both feel an increased opening deep in the pelvis. You will also have more awareness and control of pelvic floor muscles. Once you have both found this sensation of opposition in the body that creates opening, you can feel the difference in your body.

Many women use the semi-sitting position without opposition to push out their babies. However, if your partner uses opposition to maximize opening, you will not use your legs to push into each other. Instead, you will take her foot and place it on your chest between the sternum and the shoulder. A staff member takes her other foot and does the same. She presses her feet into both of you during the contraction, while she simultaneously pulls with her arms behind the knees.

NOTE: While semi-sitting is a commonly used position, especially in hospital births, this position puts pressure on the tailbone and restricts mobility in the sacrum.

HOW TO USE SQUAT POSITION WITH OPPOSITION

Squatting positions are excellent for birth. Janet Balaskas, author of *Active Birth* explains: *When the mother squats, the sacrum is free to move, allowing the...diameter of the pelvic outlet to widen by as much as 30 percent...."*[j] Many ancient depictions of birthing women show women in a squat with the baby's head emerging. Squatting makes maximum use of both gravity and anatomy to birth the baby. If your partner is comfortable in a squat, it is the optimal position for birth.

Help your partner get into any squat position in which she is comfortable. Then offer her your hands to pull on while she simultaneously presses her feet into the floor. Use your weight instead of your strength to support your partner by slightly leaning away from her. By pulling with her arms and simultaneously pressing into the floor with her feet, she uses opposition to maximize the opening at the pelvic outlet and leverage her strength.

PRACTICE SEMI-STANDING SQUAT WITH OPPOSITION FOR BIRTH
If your partner is not comfortable in a full squat, use a semi-standing squat. In drawings of tribal births, the mother is sometimes depicted as holding onto a branch of a tree while she does a standing semi-squat to deliver the baby. Stand facing one another. Hold hands and lean away from each other. Your partner then lowers her bottom as far as she is comfortable, while she pulls against you, rounds her spine, and presses her feet into the floor. Your hands provide the same dynamic for her as the tree branch while she does a semi-standing squat. Remember to use your body weight, instead of your strength, to support her. She also needs to contract her pelvic floor muscles to avoid pushing during practice.

PRACTICE PREPARES YOU BOTH
By practicing these pushing positions with your partner, you help her find that place within her where she can be an effective pusher. If you practice them once, it will guide you both when she is in the pushing phase of labor. The basic concept of the pelvic tilt combined with opposition can be used in any position. Pushing is more fully discussed in Chapter 23, along with a few more birth position options.

TECHNIQUE, PRACTICE, FREEDOM
If you try the yellow circle soft gazing and cornstarch relaxation experiments in Chapter 5; practice the breath intervention and focal techniques discussed in Chapters 10 and 11; as well as the breathing, relaxation, and preparation practices in Chapters 14–16, you will have the tools you need to respond to your partner during labor. Carter commented: *Going through the hands-on practices in your class made a huge difference for both of us. Doing it is so different from knowing it. Once my partner was in labor, I didn't have time to consider what to do. But I was able to do what was needed because we had practiced. And we both felt good about how we handled labor.*

If you practice the techniques before labor, it will give you more confidence and free you to be in the moment so you can respond to the changing needs of your partner during labor and birth.

PACKING ESSENTIALS

Below is a list of packing essentials to put in an overnight bag. Put the packed bag in an accessible spot or in the trunk of your car so it's ready to go when you need it. Your partner will also pack a bag. Confer with her so you are not duplicating. If you are planning a home birth, gather appropriate items and have them close at hand.

PACKING LIST

- Insurance card and any admissions paperwork
- Small amount of money and change for parking, vending machines, etc.
- Birth plan, if your partner made one
- Eyeglasses, if you wear them
- Cell phone or phone card with essential phone numbers of family and friends
- Camera/video camera with a memory card and batteries or film
- Music CDs to play during labor
- Toiletries like toothbrush, toothpaste, deodorant, and razor
- Protein bars
- Large container of water or tea
- Green drink or protein powder to mix with water or tea for sustained energy
- An apple
- Sweater or lightweight jacket
- Change of clothes
- Slippers
- Robe—if you plan to spend the night in the facility after the baby is born
- Bathing suit—so you can get in the shower with your partner
- Plastic bath pillow
- Nasal spray decongestant
- Lip moisturizer
- Handgrips (refer to section on handgrips)
- Hot packs
- Massage oil
- Small hand-type massager
- Extra pillows (the hospital is often in short supply)

CHAPTER 16

- Your copy of *Fathers at Birth* (Check out the appendices at the end of the book for easy reference.)

WHAT TO WEAR
- Loose, comfortable clothing (You don't want to be restricted in your movement.)
- Comfortable, supportive shoes

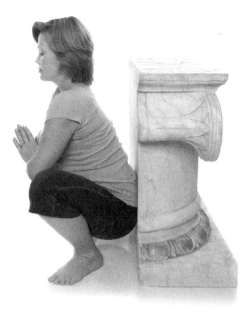

Figure 16.1 Squat position is excellent for pregnancy and birth.

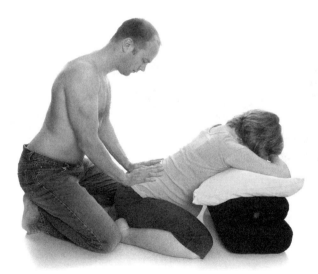

Figure 16.2 Supported all fours position helps to relieve back pressure during pregnancy as well as labor. This is a great position for you to provide counter-pressure for your partner's back.

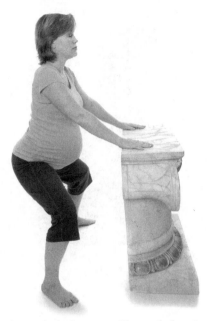

Figure 16.3 Standing pelvic tilt helps to relieve abdominal and lower back pressure.

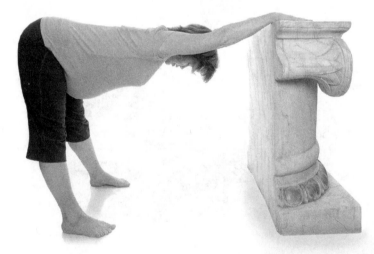

Figure 16.4 Supported back-stretch is also a good position for you to provide counterpressure for your partner's back.

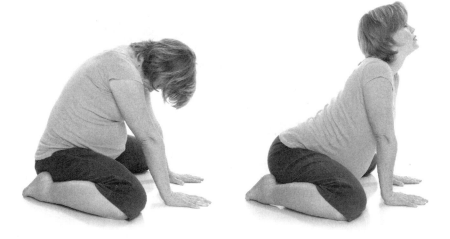

Figures 16.5 and 16.6 Frog position is soothing to many pregnant and laboring women and helps to reduce lower back and abdominal pressure. You can also provide counterpressure for your partner's lower back in this position.

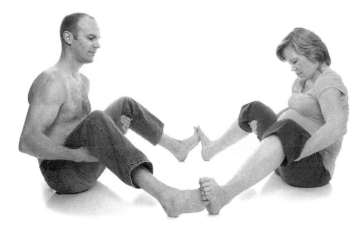

Figure 16.9 Practice the push-pull technique in semi-sitting to help your partner discover the benefits of opposition, which maximizes pelvic opening during birth.

143

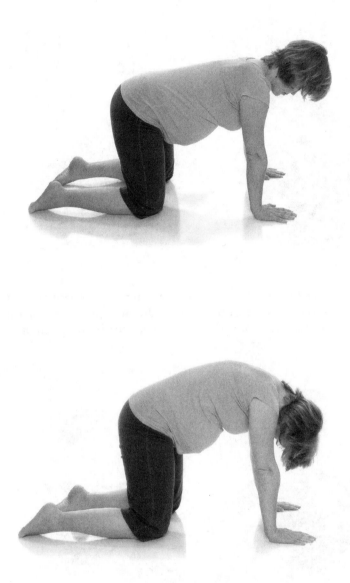

Figure 16.7 and 16.8 In the traditional all-fours position, your partner gets on her hands and knees, which gets the weight of the baby off her spine. She can also combine this position with pelvic tilting.

PART FOUR

LABOR AND BIRTH

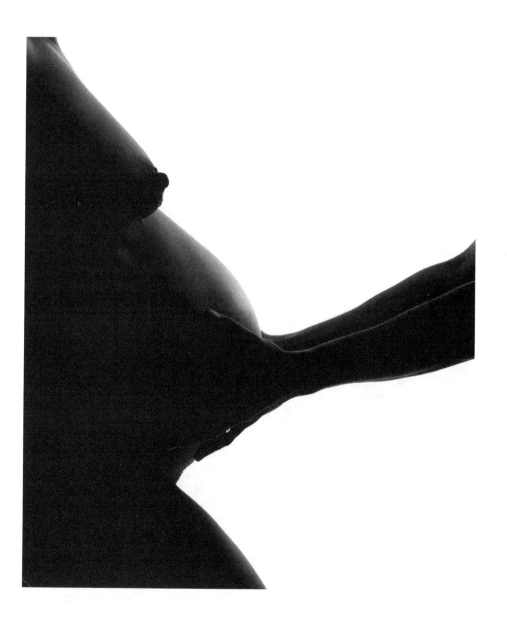

CHAPTER 17
LABOR BEGINS

EARLY LABOR

This is the moment you have been waiting for. All the months of preparation, all the images and visions of how it would come about, all the moments of wondering if the next moment will be the one you get a call or nudge in the middle of night. Suddenly it all comes together, and the time is now. The time has come to put practice into action. Labor is going to continue until the baby is here. It's time to use what you know to help bring your baby into the world.

Early labor can last from one to twelve hours (or more). You need to remain flexible to operate within the time span. You will tend your partner and oversee her needs. Provide food and liquids; make needed phone calls; gauge weather and traffic; hold and comfort your partner; track contraction intervals; load the car; massage your partner; get hot packs; encourage her to breathe and focus; track contractions again. It is starting to feel like it's up to you, so remind yourself that you are the supporting cast.

Early labor can be a special and intimate period. Do what you can to relax, enjoy, and even indulge it. Before labor begins, spend some time visualizing—choreographing in your mind what you have to do to ensure a smooth transition from early labor at home to the more advanced active labor at the birthing facility of your choice.

You are setting the tone for the rest of labor and delivery now. With all there is to do, with all the uncertainty you now face, it is easy to kick into hyper-manager mode. Don't. The mountain is not a hyper-manager. So, the most important thing to do is to take a moment to compose; to find your mountain space…and begin.

This chapter provides information you need for early labor. It includes signs your partner may exhibit, how you can assist her, and several real-life early-labor stories that illustrate the range of experiences for different couples.

SIGNS THAT YOUR PARTNER MAY EXHIBIT IN EARLY LABOR
- Burst of energy

- A pattern of emerging waves (contractions)
- Low and persistent cramping
- Lower backache or back pain
- Several soft bowel movements
- Mild flu-like symptoms
- Persistent waves (contractions) that become closer together and increase in intensity
- Bloody show or blood-tinged mucus
- Leaking of amniotic fluid (This can be a slow leak—your partner may initially think she is leaking urine. Or it can break with a gush.)
- Varying and changing emotions—elation, fear, excitement, doubt, etc.
- Nausea—especially if she smells food
- Vomiting—this is often a sign that labor is advancing
- Becoming less social (As labor progresses, contractions occupy her attention during the waves, as well as between them. She becomes less aware of what is going on around her.)

WHEN TO LEAVE FOR THE BIRTH FACILITY

Once your partner's labor begins, the big question a lot of men have is: *How do I know when I need to take my partner to the birth facility?* Observe your partner's behavior and time contractions. When she quits being social and her focus between contractions is more about labor and less about what is going on around her, it is likely time to move to the birthing facility. At this stage, she is able to walk and talk between contractions, but she may be spacey.

Be sure to consult with your medical caretakers and get their specific instructions as to when they want you to arrive at the birth facility. Even though many suggest leaving when contractions last sixty seconds and are five minutes apart, yours may have different instructions for you. Be sure to consider road conditions, traffic, and distance. If you are having a home birth, you do not need to concern yourself with when to leave. However, you need to make sure the medical practitioner arrives in plenty of time to attend your partner.

Some factions in the birthing community advocate laboring at home as long as possible to limit the medical community's opportunity to adversely affect labor. But some find that late labor flows with more ease if the mother arrives at the birthing facility before active labor requires all of her resources. That way she has time to settle in before the thick of deep active and transition labor. She is free to concentrate on the most challenging part of labor without the disorienting shuffle of having to change locations. It's kind of like stopping to set up camp before dusk.

Below is a checklist of markers to help you determine when to leave for the birth facility. If you are having a home birth, adjust the checklist to your situation.

CHECKLIST TO HELP YOU DECIDE WHEN TO LEAVE—
- Has she been in contact with her doctor or midwife? What have they told her?
- How close is the birth facility?
- How are current road conditions and traffic?
- Does she have a history of any physical problems that could affect the birth?
- When did her labor start? If this is not her first baby, how fast was her last labor? Usually each successive labor is shorter, but not always.
- How close together are the contractions, and how long are they lasting? You will need to time a series of five consecutive contractions.
- Once you have timed contractions and observed your partner's behavior, check with your practitioner for specific instructions. Even though many suggest leaving when contractions last sixty seconds and are five minutes apart, yours may have different instructions for you. Be sure to consider road conditions, traffic, and distance.
- If attendants are driving to your home for a home birth, you need to be aware of road conditions and traffic so they arrive in plenty of time.
- Is your partner easily managing contractions, or are they strong? Is she able to talk and move around between them, or is she grimacing during the contraction and becoming less social between them? Is she talking between contractions? If not, get going-or if you are having a home birth, let your practitioner know she needs to come immediately.

- Is your partner vomiting? Vomiting can be a sign that active labor is progressing. If she starts vomiting, contact your practitioner and be prepared to leave.
- Is she leaking amniotic fluid? Let your practitioner know if it breaks with a gush, and be prepared to leave.
- Don't neglect to load the car—the earlier the better.
- Contact your practitioner with any concerns.

REAL-LIFE EARLY-LABOR STORIES

Early labor experiences vary widely. Often the nesting instinct is strong in early labor. If your partner is puttering around the house during early labor, working on projects to get ready for the baby, leave her be. When labor gets challenging, you will know it.

Megan talked about her need to have everything in place for the baby and the surge of energy she experienced during early labor: *When labor began, I geared into hyper mode. I bustled around the house, making sure everything was in its place. I even got on my hands and knees and scrubbed the kitchen floor!*

Other times in early labor, a woman is derailed by powerful and surging emotions. Molly shared how early labor struck her: *When labor began, I got this wave of sheer terror. The hugeness of labor, the risk of it all, and the changes it would bring hit me with force, and I didn't know if I could do it.*

Her husband Evan commented: *We had already been through two labors and she did fine. I didn't get why she was so terrified. But I held her and listened to her, and she was able to calm down.*

If she wants to talk, attentively listen. Let her express her feelings, but avoid the desire to *fix it*. Labor itself is huge; it marks a passage to a new way of life. At the onset, she may be struck, and even a little stunned, by some of the deeper realities of what labor is about. She may even feel sorrow as she realizes that her life and her relationship with you will never be quite the same.

Marv commented: *When I got home, my wife had this frenetic energy. She was buzzing around and I felt like I was in the way. I finally suggested going for a walk and we connected during the walk.* In instances such as this, help your partner relax and focus. This helps to ground and settle her into labor. Suggest a walk, a massage, or whatever you think would interest and focus your partner.

Leigh-Ann shared that when her second labor began, she didn't realize she was in labor: *I knew I was having these light waves, but they didn't stop me, so I didn't think much of it. I went for my scheduled checkup later that day, and I was at five centimeters. They sent me right to the hospital. But at that point, I couldn't even tell for sure I was in labor. I was at seven centimeters before it felt like unmistakable labor.*

Her husband Zeke shared: *I went to the checkup with her. We live forty miles away, and the roads were icy. No wonder they wouldn't let her leave. I had to take our son to a friend's house, drive home and get our stuff, and get back. I was worried about getting back in time, but I did.*

Kristin shared how she and her partner were connected and focused during early labor: *My husband massaged my feet while we drank tea and talked. I did a lot of positions and pelvic tilting and he massaged my lower back and used hot packs. It set the tone for the whole labor.*

Each labor is unique. Each woman is unique. There are no prescriptions. Your partner may experience a wide range of emotions in early labor. She may experience excitement, compulsive behavior, denial, fear, doubt, anxiety, terror, elation, stillness, and more. Let her express, and be supportive. Hold and protect the space like a warrior and give your partner the freedom to be fully where she is.

WHAT TO DO IF LABOR STARTS IN THE MIDDLE OF THE NIGHT

If your partner wakes you up in the middle of the night and thinks she is in labor, what should you do? Often she has gotten up to use the bathroom and something is distinctly different. She may have cramps or a backache. A rhythm of waves is emerging and she wants you to know. This could be the beginning of labor.

If the waves are rising and falling, but not yet gripping, it is wise to get as much rest as possible. Not knowing how long labor will last, you both need to be as rested as possible to deal with the hard work ahead of you. One way to help your partner rest is to keep your body close to hers. Lie in bed together, and either cradle her or lie back-to-back so she can lean into you for support. Your presence and warmth is reassuring. Rest or sleep as long as it works. (*see* **Figure 17.1**)

Your partner will not sleep through active labor, so you don't need to concern yourself while you rest. However, during transition labor, it is possible your partner will drop into sleep. Allison shared: *Deep labor was so demanding and exhausting that it took every ounce of energy I had to get through each contraction. After a contraction, I would be so spent that I dropped immediately into sleep. When I woke up, I was into the next over-my-head, can't-imagine–it-could-be-this-powerful contraction. My husband told me later that the contractions were only about thirty seconds apart, and I was falling asleep between them. Can you believe it?*

Allison's experience demonstrates how rigorous labor can be, how much energy is expended, and how important it is for you both to be as rested as possible. If sleep and rest are not working, hold her and talk quietly. Suggest a bath or a shower. Get fluids for you both. Time contractions. Be the mountain.

DRINKING AND EATING DURING EARLY LABOR

Before labor begins, ask your medical practitioners what foods they recommend for early labor. They often suggest foods like fruit, crackers, cereals, toast, soft-boiled eggs, broth soups with vegetables, etc. Plain or vanilla yogurt is also an excellent early labor food, because it provides protein and is easily digested. During early labor, if the mother has an appetite, she should snack and take fluids regularly.

Once early labor is progressing, your partner may be too nauseated to eat, but hydration is important. Offer fruit juice, green drinks, or herbal teas with honey, and encourage her to drink. Make sure to take care of yourself by eating nutritious food with a good portion of protein. If you get fatigued because of hunger, it impedes how you attend your partner. If you don't want to cook, or if the smell of food nauseates your partner, consider a protein drink with yogurt or hard-boiled eggs with some fruit and a slice of toast.

DETAILS YOU NEED TO TEND TO IN EARLY LABOR

- Take care of personal needs—shower, dress, eat, etc.
- Load the car with the packed bags to take to the birth facility, or if you are having a home birth, make sure the essentials you will use during the birth are at hand.
- Make pertinent phone calls.
- If you have older children, arrange to have them cared for so your attention can be exclusively on your partner.
- Relax your body, tend your breath, and focus your mind.
- Buffer her space, minimize distractions, and free her to focus on her contractions once they start commanding her attention.

- Time a series of five consecutive contractions. You will likely do this a few times. Chart the progress.
- Lovingly attend your partner by using any of the suggestions listed below.

HOW TO ASSIST YOUR PARTNER IN EARLY LABOR

Below is a list of suggestions to assist your partner in early labor. Use what works.

- If she has a need to finish some important tasks to prepare for the baby's homecoming, help her finish whatever it is she needs to get done—or stay out of her way if she doesn't want help while she finishes whatever it is.
- Encourage her to rest, especially if it is the middle of the night.
- Offer fluids and light snacks. Encourage her to drink.
- Draw a bath for her. Bring her something to drink while in the tub.
- Take a shower together. Slow dance in the shower.
- Take a walk outside if the weather is pleasant.
- Let her talk. Listen to her without judgment or criticism.
- Use massage anywhere she finds it comforting—lower back, shoulders, feet, etc.
- Provide counterpressure on her lower back—if it feels good to her.
- Use hot packs on her lower back or anywhere it feels good to her.
- Encourage her to focus, breathe, and relax. (You need to focus, breathe, and relax too.)
- Encourage supportive early labor positions: side-lying for rest, squat, all-fours positions, rocking on a ball with pelvic tilting, frog position, slow dancing, and spinal stretch.
- Encourage her to use the cervix-breathing as a focal point. (See Chapter 11 for Cervix-Breathing for Early Labor description.) She may want to use tailor-sitting position while she focuses on the cervix and breathes into and out of it. She may want support in tailor sitting. (*see* **Figure 17.2**)
- Use the dive-into-pressure technique by encouraging her to take her awareness into the pressure, and breathe into it

and through it, softening and releasing it with the breath (See Chapter 11 for description.)

- Be tuned into your partner so you can monitor when to leave for the birthing facility or when to contact your medical practitioner to come to your home for a home birth.
- Do whatever makes your partner feel cared-for and supported. Her emotions affect how she responds to labor, so nurture her!
- Be her mountain.

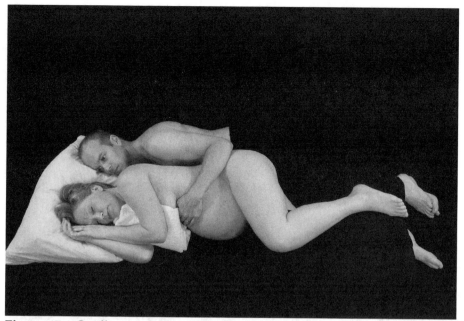

Figure 17.1 Cradle your partner while you both rest until the waves become stronger.

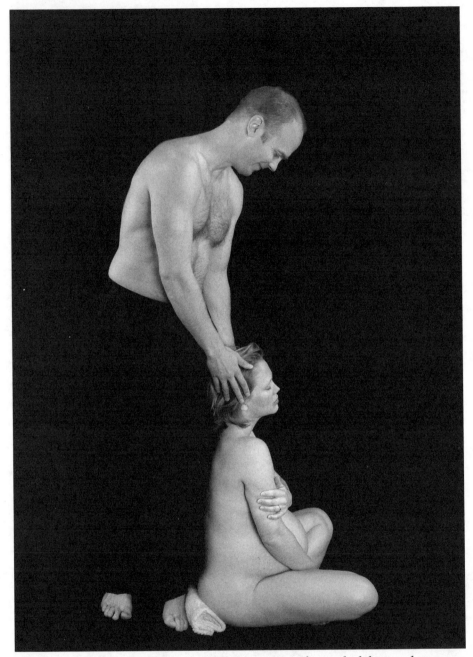

Figure 17.2 Tailor sitting is an excellent position for early labor and you can easily provide support for her in this position. She can also combine this position with cervix-breathing.

CHAPTER 18
What to Do if the Baby Arrives Unexpectedly

THE SPEEDY DELIVERY
In the vast majority of cases, labor is long enough and you are able to read the signs clearly enough to get to the birth facility before the baby arrives. For a home birth, you are usually able to contact the practitioner in time to come to your home. However, there are those rare incidences when the baby comes rapidly and unexpectedly, and you are the only one there to help your partner deliver her baby.

Here is Scott's story about what he called the "speedy delivery":
My wife phoned me at work to tell me she was in labor. She didn't sound like things were progressing too fast, but my office is more than an hour's drive from home, so I left. When I got home, she was moaning on the sofa and her contractions were coming fast. I wanted to get her to the hospital right away. But she had to make a bathroom trip, so I helped her into the bathroom. When I went to check on her, she told me the pressure was really bad. Before either of us knew it, the baby's head started coming out. I had this moment of terror thinking the baby might be born in the toilet. I picked her up and carried her to the bed. She did two maybe three pushes, and the baby was out.

If your baby arrives unexpectedly, know that most births that happen rapidly are uncomplicated and straightforward. Trust body wisdom. Birth is completely natural. (If a taxicab driver can assist a woman to deliver her baby, so can you.)

WHAT TO DO IF THE BABY IS COMING NOW
Do the following to assist your partner:
1. Make a phone call for medical assistance or dial 911—if there's time.
2. Help your partner get into all-fours position while you gather things together. This will help to slow labor.
3. Grab soap, a stack of washcloths and towels, a pan with hot water, olive oil, and blankets, and bring it all with you, placing it near your partner.
4. Wash your hands thoroughly.

5. Dive into your breathing to focus and calm. You need to concentrate and be clear.

6. Help your partner to get into a comfortable, supported position. (Squat position is optimal.)

7. Unfold four towels, lay them on top of one another, and place them underneath your partner's pelvis.

8. Take a warm washcloth with soap and water. Gently wipe the vaginal area from front to back. Take another washcloth with warm water and wipe from front to back to rinse.

9. Once you see the crown of the baby's head, massage oil into her perineum and use a warm washcloth as a compress, or your hands to support the bulging perineum. This helps to reduce or eliminate tearing.

10. Encourage your partner to relax her face and breathe diaphragmatically between contractions. If she relaxes between contractions, body wisdom will better guide her during the pushing contractions. Encourage her to breathe slowly and take her time.

11. If it is an exceptionally fast delivery, she may only push a few times.

12. If your partner passes feces, which is likely, use a warm washcloth, wipe away from the vagina, and remove it.

13. As the baby's head emerges, support the mother's perineum.

14. After the head comes out, support the baby's head by cradling it in your hand. The baby may have the umbilical cord wrapped around his neck. Most of the time you can safely leave the cord in place. If you need to loosen it, continue to support the baby's head with one hand while you gently loosen the cord with the other hand. Do not use force to pull the cord. If it is tight, you will have a chance to loosen it once the tension on it lessens.

15. After the head emerges, it may take a few contractions for the shoulders to rotate into position. Support the baby's head and be patient. You can also use this time to take a warm washcloth and wipe the mucus away from the baby's mouth and nasal passages.

16. If the baby doesn't glide out in the next few contractions, let the weight of the baby's head hang down while you support the head with your hand. The weight of the baby's head en-

courages the shoulders to release so the baby can be born. Don't pull on the baby. Let your partner's body do the work.

17. If the baby's shoulders still do not release, have your partner get onto her hands and knees. This is called the Gaskin Maneuver, named after Ina May Gaskin, who has used this position to successfully help women deliver babies whose shoulders would not deliver.

18. Once the baby is born, if the baby is not yet breathing, do not panic. The baby continues to receive oxygen through the umbilical cord for several minutes after birth. Use your mouth to gently suck the mucus and fluid out of the baby's nasal passages and throat.

19. Then gently free the umbilical cord, if it is encircling the baby. Don't pull on the cord, as this could cause additional bleeding in your partner's uterus. Give the baby to the mother to hold, nurse, or massage.

20. Get blankets and cover mother and baby. Keeping them both warm is very important.

21. Encourage your partner to nurse the baby; it will help the uterus contract, the placenta to disengage from the womb, and prevent unnecessary bleeding in the mother.

22. Do not clamp or cut the baby's cord. Wait for assistance to come. Initially, while the placenta is still attached to the mother's uterus, the cord will continue to supply oxygen to the baby. The cord will stop pulsing and clamp on its own as the placenta detaches from the uterus.

23. Enjoy these exceptionally intimate first moments of your baby's life with your partner.

24. If your partner delivers the placenta before assistance comes, collect it and put it in a bowl. The medical caretaker will want to examine it to make sure all of it has passed. Keep the bowl close to your partner and baby as the baby is still attached to the placenta via the cord.

25. Once the mother and baby are warm and stable and the placenta has been delivered, remove the stained and wet towels and put down fresh towels until your partner can get up. Get your partner some sanitary pads.

26. Offer your partner fluids. She may need assistance to use the restroom.

27. Take more time to enjoy and share the wonder of your new baby with your partner.

28. Appreciate the contribution you made. Tell the new mother what a great job she did.

WHAT ARE THE MOST ESSENTIAL STEPS YOU NEED TO TAKE?

If the baby is coming rapidly, like the delivery Scott recounted in the story above, you won't have time to do everything on this list. If that's the case in your birth, do the most important steps:

1. Help your partner into a supported, comfortable position.
2. Wash your hands, if there's time.
3. Dive into your breathing to focus and calm. You need to concentrate and be clear.
4. If the baby's head is already emerging, support your partner's perineum while the head is being delivered.
5. After the head emerges, it may take a few contractions for the shoulders to rotate into position to be born. Support the head. Don't pull on the baby. Let the mother's body do the work.
6. Once the baby is born, gently free the umbilical cord. Don't pull on the cord.
7. Give the baby to the mother to hold or nurse. After the baby is born, cover the mother and baby to keep them warm and make a phone call for medical assistance. Then refer to the list above and do whatever applies in your situation.

CUTTING THE CORD

If for whatever reason assistance cannot get to you, there is no hurry to cut the cord. You can wait several hours. As a matter of fact, some factions in the birthing community prefer to leave the cord attached to the placenta until it separates on its own. This is referred to as *Lotus birth*; the cord separates from the placenta around three days after birth.

If you decide to cut the cord, consult with your medical practitioner by phone to get details on tying and cutting the cord. Your medical practitioner may advise you to use tough thread or string to tie off the cord. If you do tie and cut the cord, sterilize the scissors and thread or string by boiling in water. Thoroughly wash your hands and allow the utensils to cool. Wrap the thread around the baby's cord about 1¼ inch (three or four centimeters) from the baby's belly. Tie securely—the string needs to stay on for a few days. Then cut the cord. Consult with your practitioner for more detailed information. Make sure to get instructions for temporary ongoing care of the baby's cord stump.

CHAPTER 19

WHAT TO DO AFTER ARRIVING AT THE BIRTH FACILITY

Once you arrive at the birth facility, your goals are to check in, assist your partner to transition into her new environment, help her get settled and comfortable, familiarize yourself with the surroundings, and set the tone for labor. If you are having a home birth, your goals are to eliminate distractions and make the environment conducive to the work of labor. Below is a to-do checklist for the birth facility. If you are having a home birth, adjust it to your needs.

CHECKLIST WHEN ENTERING THE BIRTHING ROOM

- Before you enter the facility, gather **required check-in information,** identification, insurance information, the packed bag of essentials, etc.
- Request a room with a bathtub as you are checking in. Some hospitals and most birthing centers are equipped with bathtubs in every room. In that case, this point is moot.
- Your partner may be taken right to the room, but you may be required to register at admissions. Most hospitals have a pre-registration process that either eliminates this step or minimizes the time needed for registering.
- Once you enter the room, help your partner **get physically comfortable in her new surroundings.** She may want to sit in a rocking chair, squat, or get on her hands and knees, or she may prefer to lie down. She may also need time alone in the bathroom.
- Once your partner is comfortable, **make another trip to the car,** if needed, to get whatever you may have left behind.
- **Locate the small, semicircular vomit pan** in the bedside table and place it on top within easy reach. If you need it, you won't have time to look for it. Some facilities are now equipped with plastic bags instead of vomit pans.

- **Locate the cabinet in the room with extra towels, washcloths, and blankets.** You may need to request extra blankets to use to support your partner's alignment, as well as for warmth.
- **Request an extra pillow or two.** You will use them to support your partner during side-lying position, etc. (Ask for the pillows and blankets at the same time.)
- **Locate the dirty-linen container.** You will throw washcloths and towels in it after bathing, showering, vomiting, etc.
- **Provide or request fluids for you both.**
- **Request a birthing ball.** It's easy to roll around and use in any space. When your partner is not using the ball, you can sit on it and be close to her. You can also stretch your back over it to relieve some tension.
- **Be courteous to the staff.** Thank them for their assistance. A little courtesy goes a long way.
- **Dim the lights. Play music.** (Most rooms are equipped with portable CD players.)
- **Cut distractions and make the environment conducive to the process of labor.**
- If you are using a doula, she will help you do some of the above. However, she may not get there right away, and you may be the one that tends to the checklist.

CHECKLIST FOR RAPIDLY ADVANCING LABOR

If your partner's labor is progressing rapidly and there is no time to get through the checklist, tend to only the most important items. These are:

- Help your partner into a comfortable, supported position.
- Get fluids for you both.
- Get out the vomit pan—if you need it, you will need it on the spot.
- Dim the lights.
- When a nurse comes in, request a birthing ball, as well as extra pillows and blankets.

GETTING SETTLED

Once you have settled your partner and gone through the checklist, take care of your needs. Place your packed bag in a convenient location because you will be getting things out of it to use during labor.

Then take a few moments to compose yourself. This is most important, as your partner is directly affected by your level of equanimity. Do your three-step, one-minute centering practice to gauge and refine your alignment, breath, and focus. You will be more available to your partner and everything will flow with more ease if you are centered and stable.

If the staff comes to insert an IV and your partner is averse to using one or wants to delay its insertion, ask the staff: *Is there a reason we can't wait?* Then take your partner for a walk or suggest a shower, etc.

If your medical caretaker agreed to forgo the IV and the order did not get communicated, the staff will need to check with your practitioner. However, if you use an IV, make sure the fluid bag is hung from a mobile IV stand so your partner does not lose her mobility. If you are at home or in a birthing center, you will not have to deal with an IV as standard procedure.

ATTENDING YOUR PARTNER DURING ACTIVE LABOR

Once you are settled, direct your attention exclusively to your partner. Is she ready to change positions? Would she prefer to walk around the facility? From this point on, your partner and her needs and desires will occupy your full attention. Your main jobs are to be her mountain and her warrior. Monitor her breath and facial tension, and respond to her cues. You will use many of the skills you learned and practiced from Chapters 10 through 16.

Use the one-minute centering practice over and over again to maintain your vigil. When you communicate with your partner, do it from your center. Be steadfast as you support your partner to find her path through labor. Do not neglect to tend your own comfort. The more centered and relaxed you are, the more it helps your partner center and relax.

CHAPTER 20

WHAT YOU CAN DO TO HELP IF LABOR STALLS

Labor occasionally stalls. It can stall after your arrival at the birth facility, or it can stall after several hours. In either case, the frequency and strength of the contractions diminish and labor ceases to progress. If labor stalls, a couple may feel discouraged and stymied. It is important for you to remain calm, because how you respond affects how your partner responds. It is also important for you to know how to assist your partner through this period.

If labor stalls shortly after you arrive at the birth facility, it may be because your partner feels anxious in her new surroundings. She needs time to adjust and relax, and she needs your assurance and protection. She may also be experiencing fear or doubt about the whole labor process. Labor shuts down in cases of extreme anxiety. The body reacts to fear and tension by releasing adrenaline, which counteracts oxytocin (the hormone needed to sustain labor). In addition, adrenaline stimulates the autonomic system to release fight, fright, or flight reactions, which may further stall labor. Laugher is a great antidote for life's stressful situations, so keep your sense of humor.

Occasionally labor stalls after several hours. The waves may continue, but lose their strength. At this stage, it may simply mean your partner is exhausted and needs to rest. Turn off the lights, tuck her into bed, and encourage her to rest.

Below are techniques to encourage your partner's process of labor. Choose a couple of them; you won't use them all. Remain confident. The baby will come.

1. *TAKE HER TO THE BATHROOM*

    Labor can stall if the bladder is full. The simplest strategy is to suggest a bathroom trip. Let her stay as long as she wants. Provide fluids for her to drink. Remain with her and help support her position. Or if she prefers, shut the door and give her privacy for as long as she needs.

2. *MAKE SURE SHE IS WARM*

A cold body releases adrenaline, which can slow contractions.

3. *WALKING*

Walking is a recommended and simple way to promote labor. Keep the conversation light and see if you can make her laugh.

4. *OFFER FLUIDS*

Provide fluids and encourage her to sip frequently. Labor demands fluids, and in a long labor a woman can get dehydrated.

5. *BREATHE*

If she is anxious, diaphragmatic breathing promotes relaxation, which may promote labor. Use the hand-on-upper-abdomen technique to assist her.

6. *RELAX THE FACE*

Encourage her to soften and relax her face. The face is the window of the body. If the face is relaxed, the whole body relaxes, and relaxation can facilitate labor. Use a touch-and-say, lightly stroking an area she is tensing.

7. *TAILOR SITTING*

Your partner may enjoy sitting cross-legged on the bed while she talks with you and connects. She can also combine this position with cervix-breathing. She focuses on the cervix and relaxes while she visualizes breathing into and out of it.

8. *SQUAT WITH ATTENTION ON THE BREATH*

Squatting may assist the baby to move into a more optimal position, which may help labor progress. Once she is comfortable in her chosen squat position, encourage her to establish a deep, slow, rhythmic breath. Suggest she combine the breath with tension and release of the pelvic floor. Once your partner has done so, she becomes centered, calm, and focused, which may help labor continue.

9. *BALL POSTION WITH FOCUS ON MOVEMENT*

Sitting on the ball to bounce, rock, circle, or do pelvic tilts may help the mother relax and may help the baby to move into a more optimal position. She can also combine movement with the breath to increase her focus.

10. *ALL-FOURS OR FROG POSITION WITH PELVIC TILT*

An all-fours or frog position can soothe your partner, especially if she is experiencing cramping or lower back pain.

Combine it with pelvic tilting and tension and release of the pelvic floor with the breath.

11. *SHOWERS AND BATHS*

   If labor stalls in early labor, a shower is preferable to a bath, because standing uses gravity. Go into the shower with her and do slow dancing, or leave her alone to give her privacy—whichever she prefers. Encourage her to do other positions found under the shower section in Chapter 22. If labor stalls after several hours, she may prefer a bath, because she may be exhausted and need to rest. Offer fluids.

12. *TUCK HER INTO BED SO SHE CAN REST*

   If labor stalls because of exhaustion, first make a bathroom trip and offer fluids. Then tuck her into bed. Give her body lots of support, make sure she is comfortable, turn out the lights, and let her rest. You need to rest too. If the bed is large enough, crawl into bed with her. Allow your breath to become fluid and flowing. As your body relaxes, it will help your partner relax.

13. *PITOCIN TO STIMULATE LABOR*

   If you are in a hospital, your medical attendant may recommend Pitocin. If you and your partner want to hold off on using medication, be sure to inquire if there is a reason you can't wait before administering Pitocin.

14. *RESIST THE URGE TO FIX IT*

   Don't instruct your partner. Let her find her own way. Remain calm. Most of the time, labor spontaneously begins again on its own.

15. *REMAIN CONFIDENT*

   The baby will come.

CHAPTER 21
BATHROOM TIMETABLE AND FUNDAMENTALS

REGULAR BATHROOM TRIPS ARE IMPORTANT
Once active labor is under way, your partner experiences so much pressure that she won't discern bladder pressure clearly. Labor supersedes the rational perspective. Because she is in an altered state, her concept of time is altered. This is why it is your job to track time and get her up to relieve her bladder every hour. You can stretch it an extra fifteen to twenty minutes if necessary.

Track bathroom time by the clock. For example, if it is 2:00 when your partner returns from a bathroom trip, your next target time is 3:00. If you have gotten her into the bathroom by 3:20, you are within the time frame. If she returns from the bathroom at 3:40, your next target time is 4:40.

On a practical level, relieving the bladder regularly protects it from injury, may affect long-term bladder health, and reduces unnecessary labor pressure. Sitting on the toilet is an excellent position. It utilizes gravity and may help the baby move down. Since the mother must relax her pelvic floor muscles to urinate, which reduces resistance, bathroom trips can move labor along at a faster rate. You are instrumental in facilitating labor by getting your partner up regularly to use the bathroom.

IMPORTANT CAUTION: A laboring woman who is medicated should not be moved without permission from the medical staff. Consult with staff and get their assistance.

HOW TO GET YOUR PARTNER UP TO MAKE A BATHROOM TRIP
In active labor, your partner is pressed to her max. Since getting up to go the bathroom can accelerate labor and increase pain, she may resist being moved. How do you handle this? First, do not ask her if she has to go to the bathroom. It forces her to use her rational mind, and gives her the opportunity to say no. The point is you are the one tracking time, and you know it is time for her to relieve her bladder.

Second, do not give her a warning. Do not say: *After the next contraction, it's time to go the bathroom.* If you give her a warning, she may spend the next contraction dreading being moved again. This adds to her anxiety and makes the process more difficult. Remember, you have a twenty-minute leeway. If you sense she is in a hot spot of accelerating labor, delay the bathroom trip to allow her to get to the next plateau. If there is no plateau, take her after having waited for several contractions to pass.

When you determine the time has come, get close to her ear, and as a wave ends, say decisively: *Time to get up and go to the bathroom.* Immediately remove the blankets and pillows that may be in the way and help her to stand up. If she is lying in bed, she may need to sit on the edge of the bed before standing, and she may have another contraction while sitting. Help her through it before she stands up. Take your time. Tune into her needs.

If she has an IV, make sure the line from the fluid bag to the needle in her hand doesn't get caught as she gets up. When your partner gets up, the mobile IV stand needs to be close to her; you push it with you as you walk. If your partner is using a fetal monitor, unhook the wires from the fetal monitor and tuck them into the Velcro band around your partner's abdomen. If the band falls off, leave it. The nurse will put it back on later.

While you are walking to the bathroom, put an arm around your partner for support. She is likely to have another contraction on the way. Stop and slow dance with her. Gravity increases pressure, and she may get agitated during the contraction because it is powerful. She may blame you because you got her up (and you are the one who got her pregnant in the first place). These are normal feelings. Do not doubt yourself. Once the contraction has passed, continue walking to the bathroom. (*see* **Figure 21.1**)

TECHNIQUES TO HELP HER RELAX IN THE BATHROOM
The minute you walk into the bathroom, turn on the water in the sink and let it flow. Hearing running water helps relieve the bladder. In order to urinate, the mother must relax her pelvic floor muscles, but this may not be easy because contractions can be intensely painful. Keep the water flowing, and give her a lot of time. Offer fluids and

place a glass on the sink within easy reach. Turn the water off once she urinates.

If running water does not help release her bladder, keep the water running and take a glass of warm water and pour it over her inner thigh. Pouring water over the inner thigh has worked each time I have used it, but it may take a few glasses of warm water.

She will either want you in the bathroom with her, or she will want privacy. If she needs privacy, close the door and leave her be. Check in periodically. Give her lots of time in the bathroom. She may stay there for twenty minutes or more.

Laura shared: *The bathroom was one of my favorite places to labor. People leave you alone, and you can concentrate and relax. When you sit on the toilet, it opens the space low in the pelvis.* Sitting on the toilet is an excellent position for mom and baby, and for labor's progress.

BATHROOM POSITION

If she needs you to stay with her in the bathroom, let her lean her body weight into you for support. Tracy shared: *The minute I sat on the toilet, my contractions got even more powerful. I was sweating and shuddering and groaning. The contractions were so intense, I blanked out with them.*

When she is leaning forward in *bathroom position,* the weight of the head cannot be supported by the alignment of her body. Being able to lean her head and some of her weight into your body helps her relax and relieves her of the additional work needed to maintain her position.

In bathroom position, your body faces her body. Her legs are wide open to accommodate labor. Place one of your legs between her legs and one on the outside. Your position is partially to one side of her body. She leans against you for support; it is a balance between the two of you. Be sure to support her head. (*see* **Figures 21.2 & 21.3**)

Go by her cues. If she wants stable presence, be that. If she wants pressure on her back, lean over and press into her lower back with your body weight. Stay comfortable and stable, as your comfort and stability help her to be comfortable and stable.

When she is ready to leave, offer her a warm, wet washcloth to wipe off her face and hands. She may need assistance to get up from the toilet. Offer her your hands, and let her pull on them as you lean away from her to leverage support.

CHAPTER 21

CHANGE POSITIONS AFTERWARD
Your return from the bathroom is a natural time to change positions. Suggest the rocking chair, the ball, a bath, etc. Go with what your partner prefers. She may prefer to lie down. Help her get settled, aligned, and comfortable. If she is using an electronic fetal monitor, plug the two wires back into the machine. Often the monitor picks up the baby's heartbeat. Occasionally, the staff needs to come in and adjust the ultrasound device on her belly to pick it up.

MUCUS PLUG
While your partner is in the bathroom, she may pass her mucus plug. It is often accompanied by a bloody show. Let the attendants know if your partner has a bloody show or is passing blood-tinged mucus.

DO I TAKE MY PARTNER TO THE TOILET IF SHE IS IN THE BATH-TUB?
Most women do not want to be disturbed by getting out of the tub to urinate. If your partner is in the bathtub, run the water in the tub and it will often cue her to urinate. Let some water out and add fresh. If she doesn't urinate, take her when she gets out of the tub. However, some women prefer to get out of the bathtub and use the toilet. Go with what your partner wants to do.

YOU CAN ASK FOR ASSISTANCE
If you have doubts about taking your partner to the bathroom, ask for assistance. An attendant can assist the first few times until you feel confident, or you may choose to have someone assist you each time. Work from where you are comfortable.

HOW TO ASSIST YOUR PARTNER IF SHE VOMITS
Although not every woman vomits, it is a characteristic component of many labors. Because the mother's entire energy is needed for labor, the body cleanses itself of undigested food. After vomiting, your partner will usually feel better. In addition, some women respond to the intensity of transition labor by vomiting.

Occasionally, a woman vomits several times. On rare occasions, she continues vomiting past the clear fluid, and vomits bile. Let the staff know if your partner vomits bile. However, beyond that, it is your

174

job to shield her from your doubts or concerns. Once your partner is engaged in pushing, nausea and vomiting usually cease.

If your partner gets nauseated during labor, locate the semicircular vomit pan or bags (which you may have already gotten out) and place nearby. If you are at home, use a bowl. Get some towels and washcloths and lay out a towel close to her. When she vomits, put the vomit pan next to her mouth, support her head, and catch all that you can. The towel is there to catch anything that doesn't make it into the pan. After she vomits, throw the towel into the laundry bin, dump the pan's contents into the toilet, rinse the pan, and wash your hands. Give her a warm, wet washcloth to wipe off her mouth and face. Offer fluids. Keep the vomit pan nearby, as she may need it again.

If this sounds unappealing, let an attendant handle it. Do not judge yourself. All she really wants is your stable presence. If this kind of stuff unnerves you, call the staff or ask another attendant to deal with it.

WHAT TO DO IF THE PAN WAS NOT IN PLACE

Sometimes the vomit ends up on the bed or wherever. If this happens, offer a warm washcloth so she can wipe off her mouth. Take towels and wipe up. Drop the dirty towels into the laundry bin in the room. Wash your hands. Take clean towels and place them over the area. Offer water.

You can also call the nursing staff or ask another attendant to clean up. Occasionally, the nursing staff changes the sheets. That's great if it happens. But if the staff doesn't change the sheets, try not to be concerned. The towels covering the area are adequate for now. And rarely does it concern a woman deep in labor.

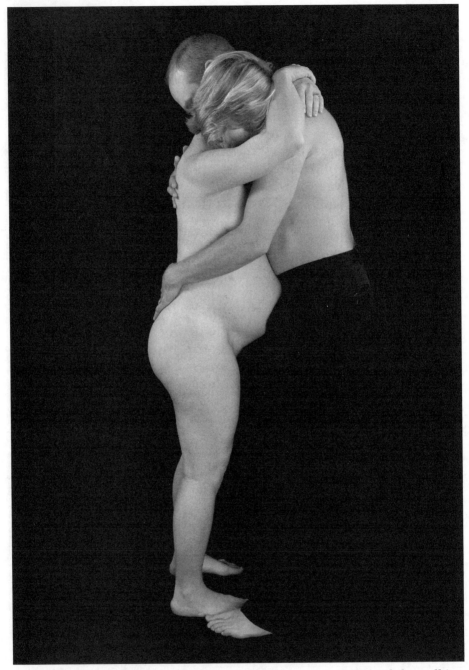

Figure 21.1 Use slow dancing position during a contraction while walking to the bathroom. Slow dancing is also a great for early labor, standing in the shower with your partner, etc.

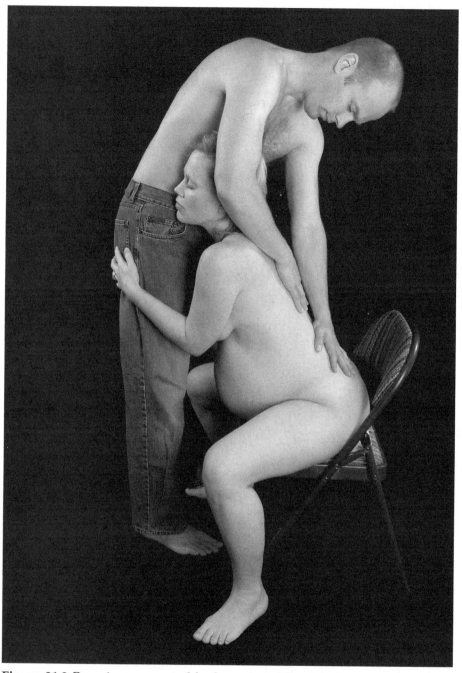

Figure 21.2 By using supported bathroom positions, you can provide additional support for your partner and also provide counterpressure for her lower back, if it comforts her.

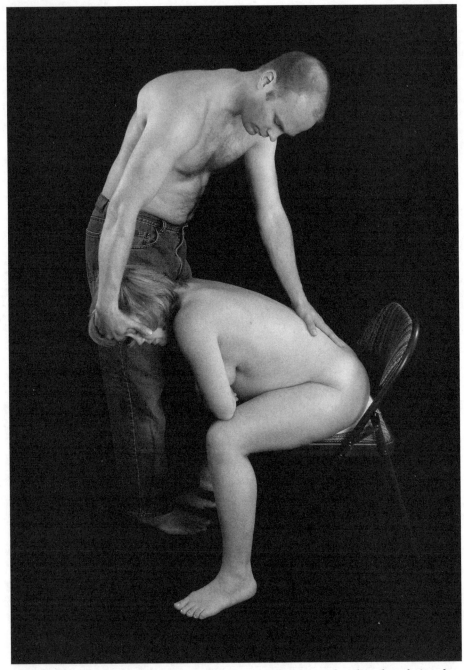

Figure 21.3 In this supported position, you can support her head and simultaneously provide counterpressure for her lower back, if she needs it.

CHAPTER 22
Labor and Water

WATER: THE TIME-HONORED REMEDY
Water is a time-honored relaxation promoter and pain reliever. A shower or bath eases the intensity of labor for many women. Because water is calming and soothing, water is also a way to set the tone for labor.

BATHTUBS AND LABOR
Once your partner is in active labor, encourage her to take a bath. A warm bath promotes relaxation, and the more your partner relaxes in active labor, the more efficient and effective labor becomes. In addition, the buoyancy of water reduces the opposition of gravity, supports the weight of the baby, and reduces some pressure.

Zoë shared her bathtub experience:

When labor started getting painful, the midwife suggested I take a bath. My husband turned on the jets and sat on a stool next to me. I put my head on the bath pillow and focused on my breath, and I could feel my body let go. Because my eyes were closed, my connection to my husband was his voice. I felt like I was connected to him through this tunnel of sound. I focused and listened. If he told me to breath to his hand, I did it. If he stroked my eye and said, 'Relax your eye,' I did it. I stayed in the bath for a long time, and my husband kept the water warm and kept giving me water to drink. Then the midwife came in and said she needed to check me. I didn't want to get out, but they helped me get out. As soon as I stood up, I got an urge to push. Getting into water helped me relax and made a huge difference in my labor.

If a bath works for your partner, it can tremendously ease labor. However, some women prefer not to take a bath, and some women are unable to relax in the tub. The most valuable strategies are those that work. Don't impose an agenda.

Water temperature should remain around 96°F to 99°F, or 36°C to 37°C. Most facilities have water thermometers. If you are at home, judge water temperature by the inside of your wrist; it should feel warm, but not hot. Add hot water periodically to keep the water warm.

Occasionally, a mother stays in the tub to deliver her baby. If this is an option in your facility, your partner may make the decision on the spot to stay in the water to birth.

BATHTUB POSITIONS
SITTING
Your partner needs to be as comfortable, aligned, and supported as is possible in any laboring position, including in the tub. In the traditional sitting tub position, your partner's back and head lean against the back of the tub. The head needs support. Blow up an inflatable tub pillow and secure behind her head. If you don't have an inflatable pillow, roll a towel and place it strategically behind her head and neck for support.

She may also need support for her back. Take an additional towel, roll or fold it, and wedge it behind her lower back. Periodically, take a pitcher or a paper cup and pour warm water over the exposed areas of the mother's body, or cover her with a towel to keep her warm. However, pouring water over her or having to deal with a towel may distract her. Go by her cues. She may also get hot in the tub, and want an ice pack to put on her face or neck.

TRADITIONAL OR MODIFIED ALL-FOURS POSITION
Other bathtub options are traditional or modified all-fours positions. In the traditional all-fours position, your partner gets on her hands and knees. In the modified position, your partner rests her head on her arms in the center of the tub and sits in a modified frog with the legs wide open. Place a towel under her head for support and comfort. All-fours positions alleviate back pressure and the water supports the weight of her belly. She can also do pelvic rocking and synchronize the movement with breath to alleviate back pressure or cramping.

USE THE BREATH IN THE TUB OR SHOWER
Encourage your partner to focus on her breathing while she is in the tub or shower. Use hand-on-upper-abdomen technique, when needed. Breathe with her. Help her use sounding. Use touch-and-say to help relax her face.

SHOWERS

Not every labor room has a tub, but most have showers. Even though a shower does not reduce the opposition of gravity, warm water falling on the skin's surface is stimulating and diminishes pain levels. In addition, water and warmth soothe the laboring woman and help her relax. You may choose to put on your bathing suit and accompany your partner into the shower to support her.

SHOWER POSITIONS
SITTING ON CHAIR

If there is a shower chair available, your partner can sit down; open her legs wide; rest her arms on her lower thighs and lean over while the warm water massages and soothes her back. She can also sit on the chair backward—cabaret style. She opens her legs, straddles the chair, and places her arms on the back of the chair so she can rest her head on her arms. She can also sit up to allow the flow of water to massage her belly.

SITTING ON BALL

Balls are great because she can combine the shower with pelvic rocking, rolling, and circling. Some women get into a movement ritual on the ball and find it comforting and focusing. She can combine the movement with sounding.

SLOW DANCING

If you decide to accompany her in the shower, use slow-dancing position. Face one another and let her lean into you for support. Put your arms around each other. Use swaying and rocking movements to soothe her.

STANDING

Your partner can simply stand in the shower. She can fold her arms and let her head rest on them while she leans against the shower wall, allowing the water to massage her back.

MODIFIED ALL-FOURS POSITION

She can bend at the hip and place her hands above her knees in a modified all-fours standing position while she does pelvic rocking. (*see* **Figure 22.1**)

CHAPTER 22

A TIME-HONORED REMEDY

By encouraging your partner to take advantage of the time-honored remedy of water, you facilitate labor. A bath or shower can shorten the time your partner labors and ease pain. I have attended many labors where the woman finished the work of transition labor in water, got out of the tub or the shower, and almost immediately got the urge to push and began pushing out her baby.

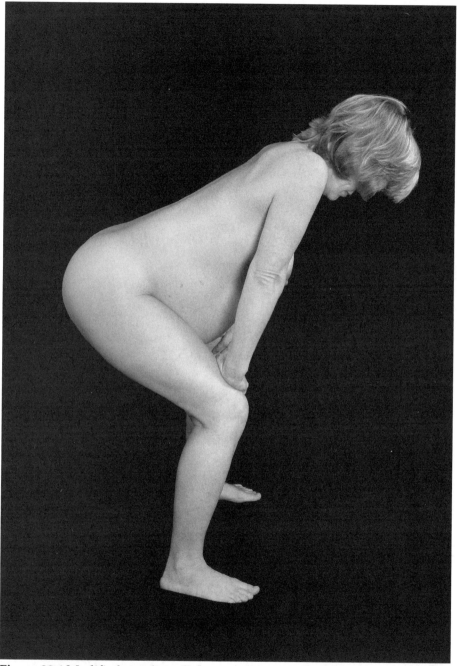

Figure 22.1 Modified standing all-fours position is a great position to use while in the shower. She can let the warm water soothe her back or you can stand behind her and provide counterpressure.

CHAPTER 23

WHAT YOU NEED TO KNOW DURING THE PUSHING PHASE
The focus of this chapter is to give you the information you need to attend your partner during pushing. The pushing phase of labor is marked by shared intimacy between you and your partner. Excitement increases as the birth draws close.

Pushing actively engages your partner. She is more alert and responsive than she was during the late stages of active labor. You may be surprised by the resolve and power your partner exhibits as she pushes. The pushing phase can be swift and straightforward, lasting only twenty to thirty minutes; or it can last three hours (or more) and be demanding and challenging.

TRANSITION LABOR: THE LAST STAGE OF ACTIVE LABOR
Immediately before your partner's pushing phase begins, she will be in transition labor. This is the shortest and most intense phase, lasting fifteen to sixty minutes or more. During this phase, your partner's body is working hard to finish the work of dilating the cervix so the baby can move out of the womb and into the birth canal.

As transition accelerates, contractions may be unbearable and continual. She may weep. She may vomit. She may fall asleep between contractions. She may doubt her ability to continue. She may demand drugs. She may think she is dying. She may be clueless she is making the last major incline of labor and soon will be pushing. She needs your rock-solid support and your full attention. You will likely be intensely involved with your partner during transition labor. It will require you to dig deep to offer her the best you have to help her through this period.

But depending on the woman and the labor, her transition labor may not look difficult. If she is on pain medication, it will not be as intense. Or, if she is not on medication, she may be in such an altered state and be so connected that she rides out the last phase with such a deep, inward focus, she transcends pain and is consciously in touch with an expanded reality and grace. Observe how intently your partner needs to focus and mentally note the pace and length of the contractions to help you determine whether she is in transition labor. Contractions may pace at about thirty-second intervals and last around ninety seconds to two minutes.

HOW TO TELL WHEN THE PUSHING PHASE OF LABOR BEGINS

At the end of transition, your partner feels pressure as the baby's head begins to move toward and into the birth canal. She may begin grunting and pushing involuntarily at the peak of her contractions. When this happens, you will know that the pushing phase is almost beginning. She may feel a powerful, irrepressible urge to push. Or she may simply be aware that an energetic shift has occurred, which she may not initially interpret as pushing. She knows something is distinctly different, but she may have a few contractions before it rationally registers that her body is pushing. You may be the first one to realize your partner is pushing. Tell her.

If you are in the hospital and alone in the room as a couple, go to the nurse's station to alert the staff that your partner has the urge to push. A medical attendant will do an internal exam to ensure the cervix is completely dilated. If she is completely dilated, the attendants will gather and give her the go-ahead to push. You will notice a difference in your partner's demeanor. Many women become exhilarated when they realize it is time to push. They become more responsive, communicative, and aware of their surroundings.

Your partner needs to be completely effaced and dilated before she begins actively pushing. Occasionally, a thick edge (lip) of cervix needs to thin and slip aside. If that is the case, the practitioner will ask your partner to hold off on pushing. Unreserved pushing through a cervix that is not fully effaced and dilated may cause swelling that could interfere with the birth.

TAKE A BATHROOM TRIP

Now is the time to make a bathroom trip. If your partner is using drugs, consult with the staff before getting her up. Getting your partner up to use the bathroom before she begins pushing serves several purposes.

First, if there is a lip that needs to slip aside, sitting on the toilet and relaxing the pelvic floor to release urine may be all that is needed to promote the cervix to completely efface and dilate.

Second, having an empty bladder during the pushing phase is important to your partner's bladder health. Your partner experiences tremendous pressure during the pushing phase. Increased pressure because of a full bladder adds unnecessary resistance, discomfort, and risk.

Third, sitting on the toilet utilizes gravity and may assist the baby to move into a more optimal position for descent through the birth canal. You tremendously assist your partner by taking her to the bathroom before she is fully engaged in pushing. If your partner has an epidural, the staff may catheterize her or assist her with the bedpan to relieve the bladder. Run the water in the bathroom if she uses the bedpan.

HOW TO HELP YOUR PARTNER AVOID PUSHING WHEN NECESSARY

If the medical attendant asks a mother to hold off on pushing during any part of the pushing phase, the mother can do so by simply keeping her breath flowing. However, for some women, the urge to push is strong and they need assistance to avoid pushing. If your partner is holding her breath or grunting, she is involuntarily using the breath and abdominal muscles to push.

To help your partner avoid pushing, encourage her to keep her mouth soft and make a *haaaa* sound with the exhalation. The *haaaa* sound keeps her jaw and throat open, which prevents her from closing off the vocal cords and using her strength to push. She can also slowly pant, sounding like this: *Haa, haa, haa.*

To further assist her, hold your finger several inches in front of her face to give her a focal point. Ask her to use a soft gaze to keep her body soft. Use a touch-and-say at the eye to help her relax. Your assistance to help her refrain from pushing when needed is important because her urge to push may be almost irrepressible.

OCCASIONAL RESTING PHASE

Occasionally, the second stage of labor starts with several pushing contractions, and then contractions stop. Contractions may skip a few beats, or they may come to a standstill for as long as thirty minutes. If this happens, the mother and staff may get anxious. However, this is a normal occurrence for some women, and is called the *resting phase*.

Sheila Kitzinger, a British author and speaker on birth and breast-feeding, refers to this as the "rest and be thankful phase." A resting phase happens more frequently in a mother who has had previous births and might also occur if the mother is exhausted from a long labor. Her body needs time to gather additional resources for the remaining work of pushing out the baby. The baby's head may be in the birth canal, but the uterus may need to tighten around the baby's body to finish the work of pushing out the baby.

Once the mother's body is prepared, pushing contractions resume spontaneously. If your partner experiences a resting phase, she needs your assurance that this is a normal pause in her particular birth. The attendant will be monitoring the baby's heart rate to ensure the baby is not in distress. Use this time to comfort and reassure the mother. Encourage her to rest and breathe diaphragmatically. Offer fluids. If your partner does not want to rest, encourage her to move around. She can walk or get into a frog position and do pelvic tilts. She can squat, use the bathroom, etc.

PUSHING POSITIONS

Once the cervix is completely dilated, your partner's bladder has been relieved, and the pushing contractions are strong, she is free to actively push. Assist your partner into a position that supports birth. Below are descriptions of pushing positions, as well as how to assist your partner during pushing.

THE PELVIC TILT AND PUSHING

One important aspect of most pushing positions is the pelvic tilt. When the pelvis tilts, the opening of the birth canal is angled in the direction the baby needs to move. Think of how a cat rounds its spine; that gives you an idea of one technique your partner can use to help birth her baby.

USE OPPOSITION: PUSH-PULL TECHNIQUE

Opposition increases opening. Before getting into the details of pushing positions, we'll cover opposition, because your partner can use the *push-pull technique* with any pushing position she chooses. The push-pull technique creates opposition, increases pelvic opening, increases control of the muscles deep in the pelvis, and maximizes your partner's effort. If your partner's pushing phase progresses slowly, if she gets frustrated, or if she needs to increase the strength of her pushing, assist her to use the leverage of opposition.

Often the staff will not be aware of the advantage of using opposition during pushing, and you may be the one that asks them to assist you with this. The opposition technique can be used to great advantage, especially by women whose pushing stage is long or difficult. Some women are guided by body wisdom to use opposition in their births. Advantages of using opposition are listed below:

- Creates leverage and increases strength
- Widens and maximizes pelvic opening
- Enhances effectiveness of the pushing contractions
- Eliminates or lessens perineal tearing
- Can shorten the length of time of the pushing phase
- Optimal use of body mechanics and strength—less strain on the mother

However, some births are rapid, and the mother does not need to use opposition. In rare instances, the mother does little active pushing. Her position and the pushing contractions do the work of moving the baby down the birth canal. This approach works for a few, but most women have a need to work with their urge to push. They literally cannot help themselves; they must push.

SEMI-SITTING BIRTH POSITION

Many women, particularly those giving birth in hospitals, deliver in bed in a semi-sitting position. The head of the bed is raised, pillows are stacked behind the mother for support, and the lower third portion of the bed is removed so the doctor or midwife can stand close to support the vulva, perineum, and baby during delivery.

At some births, the father sits behind the mother in bed to provide support. This approach is used in some home births or birthing center births because the head of the bed cannot be rolled up. If you use this position, you provide additional support for your partner to round her spine, create a pelvic tilt, and push during the contraction. Between contractions, you cradle her as she leans her back into you and rests. This position keeps you very close to your partner, and you can help her relax between pushing contractions. (see **Figure 23.1**)

If your partner wants to use opposition in semi-seated position, wedge pillows behind her back for support and stand near her foot. Your position at her foot puts you in a great place to watch the birth of your baby. When the contraction begins, take her foot and place it on your chest between the sternum and the shoulder. A staff member takes her other foot and does the same. Lean toward her and use your body weight to provide a counterforce against her foot. Your partner presses with her feet, and simultaneously pulls behind her knees to create opposition and a wider opening in the pelvic outlet. She then uses breath, abdominals, and pelvic floor muscles to actively push out her baby. The goal is to create leverage by using the push-pull technique, widening the opening and giving her more power to push.

At some births, the woman is instructed to pull her knees up, but simply pulling her knees up decreases pelvic opening. When she uses the push-pull technique in semi-sitting position, she pulls behind her knees and presses with her feet simultaneously; this move increases pelvic opening and leverages her strength without decreasing the pelvic opening.

SQUAT POSITIONS FOR BIRTH

Squat positions are excellent for birth. (However, if your partner has an epidural or is still numb from pain medication, she may not be able to get into a squat position.) Squatting uses gravity to assist the baby in his descent through the birth canal, widens the pelvic opening, and puts the mother's pelvis in optimal position to birth. (Squat positions are discussed in Chapters 15 and 16.) Your partner can use a free-standing squat, a supported squat, or a semi-standing squat. In a supported squat, she can hold onto your hands. (Remember the image of the tree branch.) (*see* **Figure 23.2**)

You can also sit on the edge of a chair with your legs wide open while she squats between your legs for support. She can face toward you or away from you. She places her hands on your legs and leans upon them as she lowers herself into a comfortable squat. Once she is comfortable, she drapes her arms over your legs for support, and you lean forward to cradle her with your arms. Between pushing contractions, she drops to the floor, either sitting or kneeling, and leans into your body to rest.

Some facilities are equipped with birthing stools. These stools support the mother in a modified seated-squat position, and are excellent to use. Sitting on the birthing stool utilizes gravity and maximizes the pelvic outlet; your partner has the advantage of a supported squat position without the disadvantage of undue strain on her knees. If she wants to use opposition, she pulls on the bars of the seat and presses into the floor with her feet while she pushes.

If she uses a semi-standing squat, she pulls on your arms and presses into the floor to create opposition. Lean away from her and use your weight instead of your strength to support her.

If you are doing a home birth or a birthing-center birth, the midwife will often get on the floor to assist a squatting mother in her delivery, but I have never seen anyone in a hospital get on the floor to assist in a squat birth. Most women squat on the bed in hospitals.

Some hospital beds are equipped with an overhead bar that your partner uses to hold onto while she squats. Squatting while holding onto the bar is an excellent birth position because it allows the mother to use opposition. You can also hang a towel over the bar for your partner to pull on. She pulls on the bar or towel and simultaneously presses her feet into the bed to create opposition. If there is no bar, she can squat on the bed while she takes your hands to pull against. Another attendant can help support her position, if needed.

LESS COMMONLY USED BIRTH POSITIONS
Other positions occasionally used in birth are side-lying position, reclining position, and all-fours positions. Your partner may prefer to use one of these positions, or she may use them temporarily. In side-lying position, the mother lies on her left side and curves her spine to create a pelvic tilt. While she pushes, an attendant lifts and supports her leg. This position can be used temporarily if your partner needs to rest during a long pushing phase.

While it is seldom used today, lying flat on the back with the feet in stirrups used to be the most common hospital birth position. If a woman lies on her back, gravity cannot work with the contractions to help the baby's descent through the birth canal. However, a reclining or semi-reclining position is still used occasionally. Occasionally, a woman chooses this position or her doctor asks her to get into this position to do an intervention.

In an all-fours position, your partner gets on her hands and knees to birth. An all-fours position takes the weight of the baby off the mother's spine and allows her to tilt her pelvis. Some women whose baby is in a posterior position (baby's face is toward the abdomen instead of the back) find this position to be particularly helpful. However, posteriorly positioned babies can be delivered in semi-sitting or squat positions too. Between contractions, the mother rests by leaning her head and torso on pillows, or by moving into frog position.

Your partner can use opposition in any of these positions. If she uses a side-lying position, she curves her spine to create a pelvic tilt, pulls behind her knees and presses with her feet while you and a staff person each support one of her feet. If your partner is reclining or semi-reclining, she pulls behind her knees and pushes with her feet into you and a staff member, which increases power and creates a pelvic tilt. If she uses an all-fours position, she presses down into the earth with the hands and knees while she simultaneously rounds the spine and uses the breath and abdominals to press low and out.

WATERBIRTH POSITIONS

If your partner chooses to deliver in water, she can use the semi-seated position by leaning against the back of the tub, an all-fours position, or squat supporting herself with her arms on the sides of the tub. Water reduces the effects of gravity and supports the mother's perineum, which may eliminate or reduce perineal tearing.

YOUR PARTNER NEEDS TO REST BETWEEN CONTRACTIONS

Pushing is major work. Your partner has two to five minutes between pushing contractions. Help her maximize this time to release tension and rest:

BETWEEN CONTRACTIONS

- Encourage her to release the last pushing contraction with a sighing exhalation. She lets the contraction and tension wash away with an exhalation.
- Help her into a comfortable, supported position so she can relax her body.
- Help her establish fluid breathing. Breathing diaphragmatically between contractions helps her rest more deeply and balances her nervous system.
- Observe her face and help her soften it with a touch-and-say.
- Offer fluids.
- Encourage her to rest.

USING THE BREATH DURING THE PUSHING PHASE

Proper use of the breath optimizes pushing. Your partner uses breath to increase strength while she pushes, and she also uses it to relax and reconnect between contractions. When a contraction begins, assist your partner into her chosen birth position. Then cue her to use the breath to maximize effectiveness:

1. First your partner takes a deep, full breath, and releases it with a long sighing exhalation.

2. Next, she takes another deep, full breath, closes off the vocal cords momentarily, and then uses the vocal cords to release the breath in short, intermittent bursts or primal sounds through the mouth, simultaneously using the torso diaphragm, abdominal muscles, and pelvic floor muscles to press deep, low, and out.

3. She pushes in short intermittent bursts during the length of the contraction and takes breaths as she needs them.

This technique allows her to use the three energy-regulating diaphragms—the vocal cords, the torso diaphragm, and the pelvic floor diaphragm—to increase power and release her baby. Bearing down, pressing in, and tightening the muscles like the action used during a bowel movement is the opposite of the optimal movement needed to birth the baby. The idea is to let the pelvic region bulge out as the mother allows the perineum to release, stretch, and open so the baby can move through.

Attentive use of breath and position makes your partner more effective when she pushes. Measured, bursting release of the breath, along with conscious use of the three energy-regulating diaphragms (vocal cords, diaphragm muscle, and pelvic floor) is beneficial on several levels:

- First, because your partner productively works with her contractions, she pushes more effectively, which can reduce the amount of time your partner spends pushing.

- Second, because the breath is released in measured bursts, it decreases the pressure on the vascular system. This eliminates or reduces broken blood vessels or capillaries that can occur because of powerful pushing.

- Third, it reduces or eliminates tearing in the perineum and can reduce or eliminate episiotomy incidence.

- Fourth, it reduces pressure on the rectum, helping to reduce or eliminate the incidence of hemorrhoids.
- Fifth, it maintains and can increase oxygen levels to the baby.

PURPLE PUSHING

Occasionally a mother holds her breath, contracts her face, and pushes with all her might while the nursing staff cheers her on. This unreserved approach to pushing is referred to as *purple pushing* and is not recommended. You can tell if your partner is holding her breath and using all of her might to push because the eyes squeeze tightly shut, her chin juts out, her face contracts, and gets beet red. Pushing with a contracted face is less productive because the energy is drawn up high instead using the wise body energies to push low, down, and out.

If a woman holds the breath for an extended period while pushing with all her might and willpower, it increases the incidence of broken capillaries and blood vessels, perineal tearing, episiotomies, decreased oxygen to the baby, and hemorrhoids, and may slow the pushing phase. Purple pushing is risky pushing. By helping moderate her approach, you help safeguard your partner and baby. Take the following steps to help your partner:

1. After the contraction is over, cue her to take a cleansing breath and release it with a long sighing exhalation.
2. Use the hand-on-upper-abdomen technique to help establish fluid, flowing, and unrestricted breath at the diaphragm.
3. Use a touch-and-say to help release residual tension in the face.
4. Attend to her comfort and encourage her to rest.
5. When the next pushing contraction begins, help her into her chosen position.
6. Remind her to take a deep, full breath, and release it with a sighing exhalation.
7. Encourage her to take another full breath and use the vocal cords to release the breath in intermittent bursts that she can combine with primal sounds.
8. Monitor facial tension with a touch-and-say to keep her face as soft as possible while she pushes.

9. Encourage her to consciously use her breath, vocal cords, torso diaphragm, abdominal muscles, and pelvic floor to push deep, low, and out.
10. Remind her to soften her face and take her energy and attention down low to release her baby.

DON'T GET TRAPPED IN THE DETAILS

Don't get trapped in the details of all this breathing and pushing instruction. It is not up to either of you. Powerful, authoritative, and wise energies assist in releasing the baby from the womb. Go with them.

Many women experience the work of pushing and the sensation of the internal movement of the baby as it moves and rotates through the birth canal as intensely gratifying. But some women feel the sensation as painful. They may get exhausted or discouraged and need lots of encouragement. Many women need to move around and change positions. Some women roar and discover a power within they have never encountered before.

Elliot, who attended his partner while she pushed, shared: *My wife went from moaning and groaning to low-grade screaming. It got so intense. It seemed to me like she was in serious pain.*

But his wife Susan commented: *Pushing was surreal and expansive. I don't remember being in pain.*

During pushing, you will be helping your partner get into position, and you will be encouraging and supporting her through the process. But you are also there to witness, share, and be blown away by the momentous event of your baby's birth.

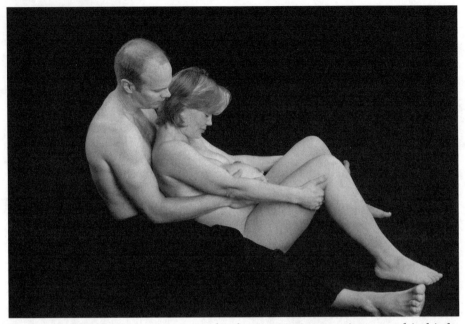

Figure 23:1 Supported semi-sitting birth position is sometimes used in birthing center or homebirths because the head of the bed cannot be rolled up. Your position behind your partner allows you to support her both during and between pushing contractions.

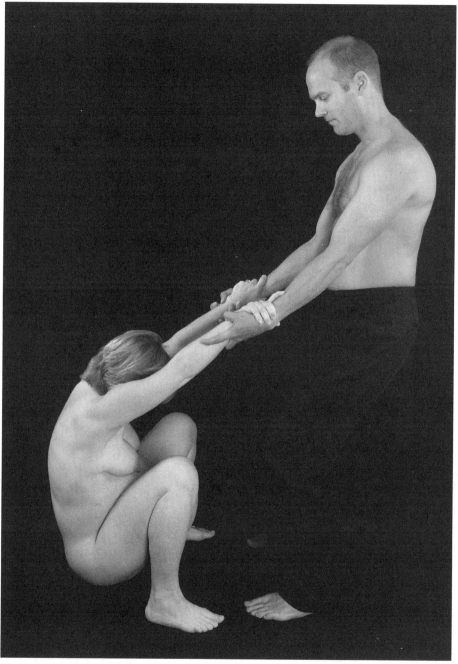

Figure 23.2 Supported squat is one position your partner may choose to use during her pushing contractions. Be sure to support her with your body weight instead of your strength.

CHAPTER 24
THE BIRTH: YOUR BABY IS BORN

YOUR BABY IS BORN
This chapter deals with details of the actual birth, some characteristics of newborns, and some of the medical routines immediately
following birth.

THE CROWNING OF THE BABY
There is great excitement when you see the top of the baby's head
pressing low in the birth canal during a pushing contraction. You will
be able to see if your baby has hair or if it is bald. Because of the
tremendous pressure on your baby's head while in the birth canal,
the top of the head may appear wrinkled. Do not be concerned; it
smoothes out once the baby has fully crowned.

First you catch a glimpse of the top of your baby's head, a piece
about the size of a dime. With each successive contraction, the size
increases until the baby's head emerges. Since birthing is a process
of waves, you may observe, like the eight-year-old boy, Sammy, who
attended his sister's birth and later commented: *Well, first the baby's
head came out, and then it went back in.* Initially, you will see the baby's
head with the pushing contraction, but during the rest between contractions the baby's head is no longer visible. Once the baby has fully
crowned, the top of the head remains visible between contractions.

When the baby crowns, the perineum begins to bulge. The medical practitioner supports the area, which helps to prevent or lessen
tearing. The caretaker may also use warm compresses or warm oil
and will likely use hands to help guide the head out of the birth canal.

If there is a standing mirror in the room, this is the time to position it so your partner can watch the birth of her baby. Often, however, the mother is so absorbed in the work of actively pushing that
watching pulls her out of the intuitive space she needs to be in to
push effectively. Go by your partner's cues.

CHAPTER 24

TRUST THE PROCESS

Birthing is an exceedingly physical undertaking. It is the embodiment of feminine power. At the core, there is no separation between the physical and the spiritual. It is one whole and holy continuum. Trust the process.

Denise related her experience of letting her body wisdom operate:

I got this primal feeling of wanting to push, and I remember thinking, 'I'm ready; let's go for it!' And my body was right there with me. I was grunting and howling and the sounds were coming out of my deepest insides. But at one point, I panicked, and I didn't think I was going to be able to do it. I got very frightened, and I thought I was going to die. I was surprised it hurt, because it didn't hurt with my first baby. Even knowing it would end didn't make it easier. My husband and midwife helped me get into a different position and the baby crowned. Then I pushed her right out and she was placed on my belly. I was in a very dreamy state. I was so in love with my baby. My husband held the baby, and we were both extremely grateful and exhausted.

You can see from the above story that your partner's body wisdom will guide her. Deep energies certainly are playing out in her body, but there are deep energies playing out in you, too. Birthing is captivating, and you will both be guided by wise energies within.

Ruth revealed how in-tune she had been with her body, but not with her rational mind, when she shared: *I was totally into pushing. It was the most intense, physically satisfying experience I have ever had. When my baby's head came out, he was faceup. The doctor remarked how well I was pushing because he had rarely seen an easier posterior presentation. I had no idea what he was saying. Right after the baby was born, the doctor told me I had a boy. When he said that, I thought, 'What is he talking about? I'm having a baby.' And then I put it together that it was a baby boy. It's obvious I wasn't thinking at all.*

Ruth's husband Roland commented: *My wife's labor had been challenging, almost grueling actually, and I expected the birth would be really challenging too. But when it came time to push, I was amazed because my wife was so into it. The only thing anyone else could do was clear the way. It was like: 'Get out of her way. She's on a mission. She's birthing her baby.' The whole thing was amazing.*

Trust your partner, trust your instincts, and go with what feels right to you.

THE DELIVERY OF THE HEAD

As the head is emerging from the birth canal, the vagina must expand wide enough to accommodate its diameter. This is the time when support for the perineum is most critical. Women may feel a burning sensation, referred to as the *ring of fire*. This burning sensation occurs in some women because of the intense stretching of the perineal tissue that must occur to accommodate the head as it moves through and out of the birth canal. The sensation may start before crowning, and be persistent, intermittent, momentary, or may not occur at all. If your partner experiences burning, you will know her tissue is being stretched to its maximum capacity to accommodate birth.

If your partner is experiencing a burning sensation, it is wise not to add additional pressure (which may cause or increase tearing) by using exertion. Cue your partner to keep the breath flowing and use a soft mouth with the *haaaa* sound. She can also slowly pant through the entire contraction with a *haa, haa, haa* sound, and let the contraction work without any additional pushing. Once the baby's head is born, the vaginal opening retracts around the neck and the burning sensation eases.

After the head emerges, the colossal work of labor is behind you both. The birth is imminent and usually occurs quickly. When you see your baby's face, the elation, awe, and grace felt in the room is palpable. Everyone is intensely focused on the birth. Vincent shared: *When I saw my baby's face, I started tearing up because I knew we had done it. We had figured it out together. And there was room for me to be human because I realized I hadn't been there in every single moment, but I had faith in my wife and it was all coming together. I knew I had helped my wife to get where she needed to be.*

The baby must now rotate (usually with support from the midwife or doctor) so the shoulders can release. One shoulder is born, then the next, and the baby slips out of the mother's body. Your baby is born!

No words are adequate to describe how you will feel when you see your infant. David expressed it this way: *Nothing prepared me for how I felt when I saw my baby. I am so thankful I was there. I wouldn't have missed it, and I feel sorry for men who do miss it. Nothing a man can ever do quite equals this experience.*

CATCHING THE BABY

You may decide to catch your baby, or you may choose to position yourself right next to your partner's head, so you can share the immediate moment of seeing the baby together. If you catch your baby, you are the one who offers your baby to your partner and places your baby on your partner's belly for her to hold. Many men find this act deeply satisfying.

Elijah shared his experience of catching his baby: *I reached down and touched his head. That made it real in a way it had not been. Then he came into the world as I cradled him, and I put him on his mother's belly. I haven't ever experienced anything so powerful.*

Collin shared his experience: *When I first touched my baby's head I thought, 'This is my daughter. This is new life coming out.' But I wasn't prepared for the fact that she would be purple and limp. Yet nobody seemed concerned. They just said, 'Put her on Mom's belly and call her in.' So I put her on my wife's belly and we started touching her and talking to her and saying, 'Come be with us.' And shortly after that she started crying and turned pink right before our eyes. It was like witnessing a miracle.*

In *Grace (Eventually)*, author Anne Lamott shared her experience of holding her son: *When he lay on my chest for the first time part of me felt like someone had given me a Martian baby to raise...and I had no owner's manual... The other part of me felt as though I were holding my own soul.*[k]

CUTTING THE CORD

Once the baby is born, the umbilical cord is clamped and cut. But many parents wisely prefer to wait until the pulsing has stopped in the cord before clamping and cutting it. Discuss this option with your medical practitioner before birth. Many fathers choose to cut their baby's cord. This act completely separates your baby from your partner's body.

Many fathers experience the birth as a disconnect from the rational, linear mind. Duncan commented: *My wife had just given birth, and I was so focused and amazed at seeing my son that I wasn't thinking at all. The doctor asked me if I wanted to cut the cord. At first I couldn't understand what he was talking about. When the doctor handed me the scissors, I was still so blown away that I could barely figure out how to get two fingers to move to-*

gether to cut the cord. I also was surprised by how firm, resilient, slippery, and rubbery the cord felt. You may be surprised to discover that you enter an altered state during the birth.

THE APGAR TEST, OTHER ROUTINES, AND NEWBORN TRAITS

Your newborn infant receives two to three *Apgar tests.* The first test is performed and recorded following birth. The second occurs about five minutes later. And the third, if performed, occurs around ten minutes later. The test measures five critical indications of vitality: heart rate, respiration, muscle tone, color, and responsive reflex to touch.

The baby is given a score of anywhere from zero to ten. Usually the second score is higher than the first. An Apgar score of three or below requires immediate intervention. An Apgar of eight or above is optimal. In addition, the baby's temperature, appearance, behavior, and alertness are monitored.

The baby is suctioned to remove mucus and amniotic fluid from the air passages. Suctioning may begin once the baby's head is delivered. Soon after birth, the baby is weighed, measured for length and head size, footprinted, given antibiotic eye drops (required in most states), cleaned up, and wrapped for warmth.

You and your partner can request that the staff hold off on these routines until the mother and you have had chance to hold the baby and welcome him or her into the world. Immediately following birth is an important time of bonding for the new family. It is best if you and your partner have as long a time as possible with your baby after birth. Your baby can be placed on your partner's abdomen immediately after being born. Your partner can hold her baby close to keep it warm, put the babe to breast, or massage the baby. You also want to hold and connect with your baby.

Your baby may be covered with a waxy light-cream-colored substance called *vernix* at birth. Vernix can be massaged into the skin or wiped off. Your baby may have a coating of light downy hair called *lanugo* on his body. Lanugo falls off within the first few weeks. Your baby is also born with a soft spot on the top of his head, called a *fontanel.* The fontanel allows the bones of the skull to compress while moving through the birth canal. The fontanel closes by around eighteen months. Your baby's head may be *molded* (elongated) at birth because of the pressure of passing through the birth canal. Within a few days, molding disappears.

The first moments of your baby's life are magical. The bonding that occurs in these first few moments between you, your partner, and your baby is intense and enduring.

DELIVERY OF THE PLACENTA: THIRD STAGE OF LABOR

Once the baby is born, the last stage of labor is the separation of the placenta from the uterine wall and its delivery (expulsion). The uterus continues contracting to completely disengage the placenta. This process normally takes seven to twenty minutes, but may take longer. The placenta is surprisingly large and meaty. It is the root from which your baby has grown. Usually the couple is so entranced by their new baby that the delivery of the placenta is not a focus.

The placenta slides out easily, usually with a gush of blood and amniotic fluid, and most women note the sensation, but find it painless. Sometimes the mother is asked to push to help deliver the placenta, and an attendant may massage her abdomen to encourage her uterus to contract. After the delivery of the placenta, your midwife or doctor closely examines it to make sure the entire placenta is intact. This is important, because if a small piece of the placenta stays embedded in the uterine wall, it can cause an infection or other problems after the baby is born.

Once the placenta has been delivered and examined, your caretaker closely examines your partner's perineum for any tears. If there are tears, or if an episiotomy was performed, the caretaker administers a local anesthetic to repair (suture) the perineum. Women generally experience the stitching as little pricks that are easily managed and most women do not find it distractingly painful. Also both of you are so captivated by your newborn and so relieved labor is behind you, that the repair of the perineum is a minor occurrence.

Some couples choose to take the placenta and have a ceremony of burying it; others are not interested. Some couples choose to have some of the blood from the cord stored; others cannot afford the storage. Some couples choose to donate the cord blood. These are individual options to discuss with your medical practitioner. These decisions are best made before birth, but you can change your mind at the time.

Due to altering levels of hormones, some women experience shaking or trembling following birth. Christina shared her experience: *Right after my baby was born, I got cold and went into shaking mode. It was like every cell in my body was vibrating, shaking uncontrollably.* This is normal for some women, and subsides shortly. Reassure her and keep her warm.

During the delivery of the placenta and the possible repair of the perineum, you and your partner will likely be holding the baby. You will want to keep the baby warm because the baby is unable to maintain his own body temperature. Your partner may also be nursing her baby. Emotions during this period are indescribable. You will just have to experience it for yourself.

CONTRACTION OF THE UTERUS AFTER BIRTH

After delivering the placenta, the uterus continues to contract and clamp down. The attendants check and massage the uterus at intervals to affirm that the uterus remains hard and contracted. This can be uncomfortable for your partner. The contracting of the uterus safeguards the mother from excessive bleeding. In addition the uterus must, in the next four to six weeks, contract back to its non-pregnant, fist-sized shape.

Some women, especially those who have experienced more than one birth, find the postpartum uterine contractions, or the *afterpains*, are as uncomfortable as labor. If your partner experiences intense afterpains, assist her by helping her breathe and relax through the contractions like you did during labor.

NURSING IMMEDIATELY AFTER BIRTH

It is wise for your partner to nurse the baby as soon after birth as possible. Nursing releases the hormone oxytocin, which assists the uterine wall to clamp down and contract. This helps prevent unnecessary blood loss after birth. Some women instinctively put the baby to the breast following the birth. Other women need reminders to do so.

Babies may not immediately suck. Some hang out by the nipple and lick it, while others latch on right away and start sucking. Nursing intensifies bonding. Encourage your partner to nurse as soon as possible after birth and support her in the endeavor. Knowledgeable attendants are present at the birth to guide your partner and answer any urgent questions regarding how to nurse.

CHAPTER 24

RELIEF, EXHAUSTION, AND EXHILARATION

Most couples are relieved and exhausted after birth, but also elated. It is a blessed time. Calvin commented on the relief, exhaustion, and gratifying mind-set he experienced after birth: *Once it was all over, it was like this veil of concern and apprehension just exploded into particles and disappeared. The weight lifted and I realized how much gravity the situation had held until I was sure my wife and baby were both okay. My sole focus as a partner had been to help my wife get the labor and delivery experience she wanted and to bring a healthy child into the world. To go through it and have it go pretty much the way we had hoped and then to have a healthy, beautiful baby at the end was overwhelming. What more could I want? After that I was exhausted. I had been up all night. But I was almost embarrassed to admit to my wife how exhausted I was because she had been the one who had done the work of labor and pushing out the baby.*

Since men are not the ones doing the actual labor and birth, they may be embarrassed to admit how exhausted and relieved they are once it is over and all is well. They may also be reluctant to admit the amount of dedication and work it took them to attend their partner. I don't think most women (or anyone else) realize the weight many men shoulder during labor and birth. What happens to a man's partner and his baby, in effect, happens to him. Gerald commented: *If you compare the amount of effort, obviously the nod goes to the woman. But I don't think anyone has any idea of the amount of effort it takes to be in a physically supportive role where you have to take action, yet be in a witness role where you have to be truly present. And the whole time I was concerned that both my baby and my wife would be all right.*

TIME TO REST AND ENJOY YOUR BABY!

The main focuses immediately following the birth are to take amazing delight in your newborn and to celebrate with your partner. Be sure to tell her what a great job she did. You may also want to make a few important announcement phone calls to family and friends. Don't neglect to care for yourself by getting some food and rest.

If you are in a hospital, there is a lot of activity and support during the birth. But once the baby is born and wiped off, has undergone the necessary medical procedures, and is swaddled, you and your partner may suddenly find yourselves alone with the baby in a very quiet room. The mother, baby, and possibly you will be staying for an extra day or two.

If you are in a birthing center, you will be leaving with your new family within a few hours. If you had a home birth, take a quick assessment of what needs to be cleaned up before extraneous attendants leave, so you can enlist their help. They may be willing to change bedding, tidy up the kitchen and bathroom, throw in a load of laundry, and take out trash. You want to ensure your partner has a comfortable and tidy environment to recuperate in.

The hours immediately following birth are extraordinary, as the whole world seems to fade away and you have this insulated time with your baby and partner. After birth, most couples are engrossed and enchanted with their newborn. It is important for you to hold your baby. Many men experience a flood of emotions when they hold their infant the first few times. Men may also be surprised by their instinctive desire to protect and shelter their new family. Take full advantage of this time to rest and enjoy your partner and baby.

EPILOGUE

GOING HOME: THE FIRST FORTY DAYS AND BEYOND

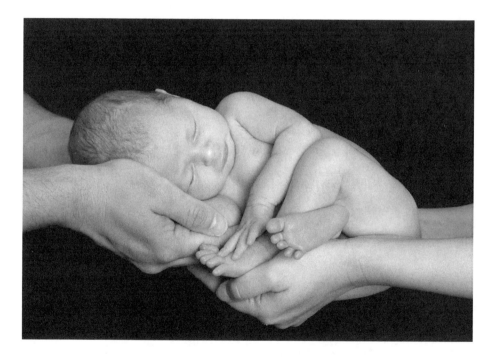

CHAPTER 25
THE FIRST FORTY DAYS AND NIGHTS

The first forty days and forty nights are remarkably special, and pass quickly. It is a time of bliss and challenge as you, your baby, and your partner adjust to your new lifestyle. It is an intensely adoring, tender, and blessed time, as most fathers find themselves falling head over heels in love. Their awareness becomes concentrated. They become captivated and take delight in every movement and sound their baby makes.

Immerse yourself in the experience. Spend time with your baby and your partner. Gaze upon your baby. Hold your baby. Be brutal in cutting out extraneous activities, and give yourself time to unabashedly and exclusively enjoy your baby, your partner, and this extraordinary beginning you share.

If this is your first baby, you will be adjusting to your new role as father and family man. If you already have a family, the whole family is adjusting to the new dynamic. Because every child is different, each child is a unique and new adventure. Give yourself lots of unstructured time to get to know your baby and adjust to your new lifestyle.

OTHERWORLDLY
Babies remain otherworldly for the first few weeks after birth. They are in the world, but are not yet quite *here*. Because your baby has just emerged from the womb, you are adjusting to the new order after birth, and so is your baby. (From here on, the masculine pronoun is used to refer to your baby since no appropriate pronoun refers to both sexes.) Before birth, your baby was held in the fetal position and wrapped securely by the womb, where it was dark and warm. Other than the beat of your partner's heart and breath, sounds were muffled.

A newborn baby has never known hunger, cold, sight, or light. Your baby was immersed in water in the womb, so he is also adjusting to the effects of gravity and air. During your baby's last few months in the womb, his movement was tightly restricted. Swaddling him is familiar and comforting, since he is used to being in a tight, warm space. Too much freedom of movement can startle or distress babies. Using a receiving blanket to swaddle your baby before you lay him down helps him go to sleep more quickly and sleep longer.

A newborn cannot support his head. When you pick up or hold your baby, support his head. But babies are resilient. You don't have to be overly cautious. Relax and enjoy your infant. William, an experienced father, said it like this: *The first baby is kind of like glass. But the second one is kind of like rubber.*

During this otherworldly phase, you will be getting to know your baby, and he will be getting to know you. When you hold your newborn, he does not yet know where his body ends and yours begins. Your body and his body are blended into one experience for him.

It is a great gift to your baby if you eliminate as many distractions as possible. But it is a greater gift to you if you eliminate distractions and focus on the job at hand—getting to know your baby and adjusting to the new order.

BONDING WITH YOUR BABY

Your infant is wired for bonding during this early phase. Holding your baby or wearing him in a soft infant pouch or sling is an easy way to bond with him and help him feel secure as he transitions out of the otherworldly phase and into this world. Wearing your baby keeps him close to your body, where it is warm and he can hear the familiar sounds of heart and breath.

Since he spent months in the womb being rocked by and listening to two continual drumbeats—the movement and sound of heart and breath—holding your baby close or wearing him in a soft infant carrier is comforting. Often babies quickly go to sleep when put into a cloth carrier. It also frees your hands, somewhat, so you can you engage in other activities while you hold your baby. In tribal cultures, babies are carried in cloth carriers for a few years. The primary way he knows your love is by feeling your and your partner's bodies holding him.

Babies like to make eye contact and gaze at faces. It's amazing how intently a baby gazes. Eye contact is one way you bond with your baby. When you gaze into his eyes, you make facial movements that respond to the movements he makes. This provides a feedback loop for him as you connect with one another. Babies also like the sound of human voices. Talk to your baby or sing to him while you hold him or gaze into his face.

Sucking is essential to your baby's emotional and physical health, and you can bond with him while you let him suck on your finger. Wash your hands and place the little or ring finger nail down on your baby's tongue. The soft pad of your finger is on the roof of his mouth. Sucking is comforting to babies. Babies also like movement; he may enjoy sucking on your finger while you walk or rock him. You can also sit on a ball and bounce him.

Touch or massage are other ways to bond with your baby. Many fathers take great pleasure in gently massaging their baby. You can also simply touch him gently, pat his back, stroke his palms or feet, or count his toes and fingers. Stroking your baby's head and patting his bottom are also soothing. Touching your baby helps him learn about his own body.

Another easy way to bond with your baby is to lie down and place him on your torso where the babe can feel the movement and sound of your breath and heart. Your baby will often drop into sleep while he is lying on your chest, and you can both get some needed rest. Your whole family can also crawl into bed together and hold the baby.

Joel remembered: *The first day our baby was home, my wife, our two older children, and I all got into bed together. We leaned against the headboard and I held the baby on my lap facing all of us. When each of us talked, the baby turned his head and gazed into the face of the person talking. You could see he was making a connection between voices that he had been hearing in the womb and our faces that he could now see. It was fascinating to watch.*

Your baby recognizes you by smell and sound, as well as by sight. His brain and nervous system continue to develop at a fast rate. It is astonishing how quickly a baby grows, learns, and changes.

BABY TIME IS NOW TIME

Babies live in the moment. They don't mull over the past or plan the future. We are conditioned to mull over what has already happened or think about what is coming up in our lives. But our babies can teach us to reconnect with the moment—where life is really happening—if we let them.

The best way to live in the moment is to simply be there and enjoy your baby. If you find yourself distracted, use the one-minute centering practice to help you be present and spontaneous with your baby.

CRYING BABIES

Babies cry. Not responding to a crying baby or frequently leaving him alone to cry for long periods is not good for his emotional health. When your baby cries, he may be hungry. If your partner is nursing, carry him to your partner. If your partner is not immediately available, hold him while you let him suck on your finger. You can also check to see if the baby needs a diaper change. If these obvious solutions don't work, movement often soothes a crying baby.

Putting your baby in a cloth carrier often comforts him when he cries. You can also swaddle your baby and hold him while you walk or dance. Make low-pitched, comforting sounds in your baby's ear while you pat his back. Bounce or rock your baby while you sing a lullaby, and let him suck on your finger. Skin-to-skin contact sometimes comforts a crying baby. Let him lie on your naked chest.

If your baby seems to be distressed because his tummy is bothering him, massage his tummy in gentle clockwise circular motions around the navel. Laying your baby on his stomach across your lower thighs and patting his back helps him release gas and soothes his tummy. These tactics often soothe a crying baby, but if none of these tactics work, put him in an infant swing or cradle. You can purchase a baby swing with a cradle attachment for newborns. Many babies go to sleep while swinging or rocking in a cradle.

Sometimes no matter what you do, your baby continues to cry. Observe your emotional state. If you are upset, it upsets the baby. The more upset you get, the more upset your baby gets, and before you know it, things spin into a downward spiral. When you are at your limit, swaddle the baby, lie him down in a safe place like a bassinette or a cradle, and take a break. Move out of earshot of the baby's cry until you compose yourself. You cannot soothe a crying baby if you are upset. Give yourself time to compose and calm.

If you get upset, know this is a normal part of being stretched as a parent. Caring for a baby is a huge job. Respect your individual, human, and honest limits without guilt. If fathers do not respect their valid limits, they may react impulsively. Giving yourself a break is healthy for you and your baby.

INTENSE EMOTION

Emotions are often intense during this period. They can run the gamut between euphoria and sorrow for you both. Your partner may weep because of ecstatic love or gratitude. She may weep because she is exhausted or overwhelmed by the phenomenal amount of work and constant responsibility. She may wonder if she will ever have her life or her body back. She may be clueless as to why she is weeping. She just needs to cry!

You cannot fix it, so don't attempt to. More importantly, don't get in your own way and take it personally. Don't vacate emotionally and put her in the position of feeling guilty or mad because she cannot, in this moment, attend to you too. Be the mountain and hold the space during the storm.

Sobbing is therapeutic. It uses the diaphragm as a plunger, which helps cleanse the mother's system. It forces the breath out in bursts, unrestricts her diaphragm, and helps release emotions. The sharp exhalations in sobbing allow the breath to flow in, which helps reestablish a fluid breath pattern. She will feel better after a good cry.

You may be able to use the skills you used during labor to assist your partner to calm. However, she may resist any attempts you make to assist her. Give her the freedom to be where she is without judgment or criticism. This is a great gift to your partner, and she will return the gift to you and the whole family when she is able.

It is important to understand that your partner is undergoing extreme psychophysiological changes, alterations, and adjustments. Her body has to adjust from a pregnant state back to a non-pregnant one. During pregnancy, estrogen levels are exceedingly high. But after pregnancy, estrogen levels drop. The modification of hormones is drastic and impacts her body, mind, and emotions.

Because of hormone alterations and the radical changes that occur in lifestyle and identity, your partner may exhibit mood swings. All kinds of powerful and opposing emotions may be surging. There may be moments when you feel like you are walking through a minefield. Remember, feminine energy is like water; it changes without warning, but it calms as quickly as it surges. Don't overreact. Use your one-minute centering practice and have confidence in your partner's capacity. The more support she receives, the more adeptly she will find her path through this time.

Give yourself the freedom to be candid about your emotions too. The adjustment after birth draws out the best and the worst in us. It pulls out what we didn't even know was in us. Sometimes it's no fun. It can be messy and muddy, and occasionally we get stuck. Be compassionate toward your partner, but be compassionate toward yourself as well. If you lose it, it's okay. In a new situation, you often must lose your balance to rediscover it. Don't make impossible demands on yourself to follow a script.

Birth and the major transition afterward push us to our limit and force us to move beyond it. They spur massive, spontaneous growth. Unconditional love opens us to the expansiveness of being, which can be quite a glimpse to take in. We discover awe, thanksgiving, and truth beyond our boundary. But they also bring into focus the more constricted aspects of our being, areas on which we need to work. This is quite a glimpse to take in too. We sit in the extremes of who we are—the positive and the negative, the expanded and the contracted. We get a wider view of ourselves. We see the light, as well as the darkness. We are humbled by both.

The experience of unconditional love you and your partner experience for your baby is a great gift. It confirms the truth that unconditional love is available and you can receive and offer it. Encountering the truth of unconditional love marks your journey toward freedom. That freedom is not the freedom to *do* what you want to do. It is the freedom to *be* who you are.

REST, QUALITY NUTRITION, AND FLUIDS

Your partner needs lots of rest during this period. If she gets enough rest, her recovery time will be quicker, and everyone in the household will be happier. Sleep deprivation in the early days, weeks, and months creates a domino effect that creates havoc in all areas. Absolutely everything will run more smoothly if your partner gets enough rest. Encourage her to nap whenever she can.

The body heals during sleep. It also takes sleep to process and adjust to the transition you are both undergoing. If your partner is nursing, it takes rest for her body to produce milk. If she had a cesarean birth, rest is especially essential to her healing and recovery. Rest is vital for the new mother. Because you are also making a big adjustment, it is important that you get enough rest too. Getting adequate sleep and rest dramatically affects how you both cope and needs to be a priority.

High-quality nutrition also needs to be a priority for you both. The mother is pivotal in family life, and her state of mind affects the whole family. Her state of mind is affected if her blood sugar gets low; then things can quickly spin out of control. Getting enough nutrition with a generous amount of protein helps your partner's blood sugar remain stable, which eases emotional swings. Good nutrition also helps your partner to recover and heal faster and increases her milk production.

Fluids are also essential for you both. Mild dehydration may not be detected, but it will affect your partner's mood and how her system operates. Offer your partner quality fluids whenever she feeds the baby. Get yourself something to drink too.

The importance of tending the basics—getting enough rest, quality nutrition, and fluids—cannot be overstated. These essentials support and smooth the transition you are all making, and help you maintain a compassionate, supportive, and loving attitude toward your partner.

WHAT CAN YOU DO TO HELP?

There is a proverbial saying in the East: The way a woman takes care of herself after a baby is born determines how long she will live. Do not take this statement literally. However, you want to contribute to your partner's receiving the best possible care and support, knowing they have the potential to contribute to her long-term emotional and physical health. It may seem to you that your partner is consumed by baby care. That's true. She is. Right now, nothing is more important than the work she is doing to transition into motherhood.

If you are able to take time off work, take as much time as is feasible. Be emotionally and physically available to your partner. The support and love you offer her contribute to her ability to enjoy and nurture your child. Your stable support provides an atmosphere in which she can recover more quickly and bond more deeply with your baby. Your attentive presence allows your partner to draw from your masculine reserve energy. She uses it to stabilize herself and the baby. This is a more valuable contribution than you know.

You can also help by taking the baby for a walk in an infant carrier or stroller. This gives your partner some downtime to do an activity she finds renewing like bathing, resting, or sharing her feelings with a close friend. It also gives you some alone time with the baby.

Do some of the diaper-changing and the baby's bathing and dressing. The first few times may be a bit unnerving, but in short order, you'll be a pro. Pitch in and help with daily chores. Run errands.

Do laundry. Prepare meals. In short, be there and do what you can to support and witness your partner's transition into motherhood as well as the beginning of your baby's life.

TAKE TIME FOR YOURSELF

Take some downtime for yourself. Schedule time to work out, have a beer with friends, go for a hike, or take a nap. Do whatever recharges you. A convenient time to slip away is when your partner has a friend or a family member with her. Tending yourself makes you more available when you are there. Make sure you are getting enough nutrition, fluids, and rest. When you tend yourself, you are better able to tend your new family.

GATHER COMMUNITY RESOURCES

Actively use any available community resources. If you used a doula, hire her to come in and assist your partner with the details of nursing and baby care. If you have family or friends willing to bring in meals or assist with chores or errands, now is the time to accept their assistance.

When family or friends come in, make sure their priority is the mother. Take care of her first. She needs to be off her feet as much as possible. Don't allow your partner to wait on them. They should be there to wait on her. They have come to help you. Of course, if your partner insists, let her do what she needs to do.

Family members who come to assist you during this extraordinarily special period need to remain focused on what they can do to support your new family. They should be there to provide assistance with the workload, as well as experienced know-how. Of course they will want to hold the baby, and most new mothers are relieved to let an aunt or grandma change a diaper or hold the baby. But some new mothers are very protective of their *baby space,* so follow the mother's lead. In either case, don't let others move in and take over the primary care of the baby. Reserve that job for you and your partner. Their job is to assist and support you and your partner as you adjust to the demands and joys of parenthood.

If you have older children, family members can be extremely valuable in caring for them. This gives your older children a special opportunity to bond with extended family. It also gives you and your partner more time for the baby during the otherworldly beginning of your new baby's life.

If you have the financial means, hire a person to come in and clean once a week or every other week for several months or longer. If your community has grocery-delivery or other delivery services, now is the time to take advantage of them. Some couples use paper plates to minimize clean-up, bring in takeout or have meals delivered, and use disposable diapers. Take advantage of whatever resources are available to minimize the workload. Do whatever you can to streamline and simplify your life.

OLDER CHILDREN

If you have an older child, now is the time to stand in the gap. (Of course, you may have several older children, but for the sake of clarity and ease, I will refer to your older child or children with the singular male pronoun.) This is a special time for a father to increase his bond with his older child. You get the opportunity to be with him at a time when he really needs you. Make good use of it.

Hold him. Play with him. Talk to him. Read to him. Feed him. Rock him. Pay lots of attention to him. Be physically present and attentive. Your older child is often content to be a special companion to Daddy while Mommy cares for the baby. For one thing, dads can be more fun than moms. A child who spends time with his father has a more developed sense of humor, which is vital to getting through life with more joy. From you, your child learns a masculine perspective toward life, which is necessary to navigating and succeeding in the world. Society does not come close to valuing the vital role of fathers.

Anticipate that your older child will be jealous of the new baby. This is normal. He may inquire: *When is that baby leaving?* He may not be able to verbally express his feelings. He may just act out. You will likely see behavior issues. Be patient and realize he is making a major change too. It takes time.

More than a few young children have been known to put a pillow over the baby's face. Be vigilant in protecting your baby, but encourage your older child to be honest with his feelings. Help him voice some of his feelings by saying: *I miss the time when it was you and Mommy and me. Do you?* Say: *Mommy is so busy these days with that new baby.* Let your child know you recognize the disruption in his life by acknowledging: *Babies are a lot of trouble, aren't they?*

Children crave love and attention from both parents. If your child refuses to leave his mother's side, but your partner needs to have time alone with the baby, take him on a special adventure. Something as simple as a walk, running an errand with you, or a trip to the local zoo can renew his sense of security and assure him he is not losing his importance in the family.

The love your partner has for her older child is unshakable. But she is currently equipped with her body and hormones to respond to the infant; the infant's ability to thrive depends on this instinctive reaction. Laura expressed it like this: *I love my older child, but I am in love with my baby.* Your older child is going to know that. And your partner may experience pangs of guilt and grief over the reality of it. However, it is how we are designed. Babies grow up, and we have to let them go. This is a step in that progression, and it is healthy for everyone.

LOWER YOUR EXPECTATIONS

In the first several weeks, you may have a flurry of people to assist you. But after that, it calms down. There is an unspoken expectation, especially in our society, that you will get back on your feet and get things back to normal—almost like nothing happened. That assumption can backfire on women, men, and families. Lilly shared: *After my first baby was born, I expected to have things back to normal in six weeks. I was shocked to discover at six weeks I wasn't even close.*

It took your partner nine months to grow the baby and it is likely to take her that long to find her stride after the baby is born. Our society does not acknowledge the great event the birth of a child is in a woman's life. It also does not acknowledge or value the monumental amount of work and dedication it takes from both parents to raise a child.

For the first year of your child's life, cut out extraneous activities and show up as best you can. Now is the time to be there. Don't miss it. Focus on your family and help establish a firm foundation.

BE THE HERO

Some say the greatest love affair, the most intense bond, is between mother and infant. You may feel you have lost the special and exclusive bond with your life partner, and you may find yourself feeling pangs of jealousy or resentment toward your infant. If you feel this way, acknowledge your honest, valid emotions. Many men feel this way, and it is a normal part of adjusting to family life. You are a true hero to your partner if you can be honest with your emotions and support her through your own struggles. As a father, you are also a hero to your child and will influence generations.

Consider that other names for God are father and mother. Many traditions teach that God is love and God is truth. It is not that God (or however you refer to it) is love in one place and truth in another. Love and truth are expressions of one absolute reality. You and your partner embody unconditional love and offer it to your child. From this perspective, to your young child, you and your partner are Mamadeus and Papadeus—God on earth, Immanuel, God with us. You and your partner are the earth, the ground that your baby grows from, but you are also a source of love and truth for your baby.

BREASTFEEDING OR BOTTLE-FEEDING:
SUPPORT YOUR PARTNER'S CHOICE

Most women choose to breastfeed (nurse) their baby, but some choose to bottle-feed. If you have an opinion on how your baby should be fed, express yourself, but do so in a way that gives your partner the freedom to find her own path. Feeding is one of the primary activities in caring for the baby. Whether your partner breastfeeds or bottle-feeds, she needs your committed support. When your partner feeds the baby, make sure she is comfortable. Wedge pillows to support her arms and head; offer fluids and nutritious snacks.

Some women have demanding jobs that prevent them from breastfeeding. Others cannot nurse because of a chronic health problem, and some need medication that is harmful to the baby and therefore nursing is contraindicated. Some women want to nurse, but have so many difficulties with it that they cannot establish the practice. Others simply do not want to nurse. They prefer to have their partners and other people involved with the feeding, and choose not to tackle a job that no one else but the mother can do.

Nursing has become such a charged issue that women who do not or cannot nurse may feel guilty or judged. Every woman has to navigate the way she has chosen. No woman should be judged for doing it the way she has to do it. Since the beginning of humankind, some situations have required that babies get milk from other sources than their mothers. If a baby is loved and nourished, that's all that matters. Everything else pales by comparison.

WHAT YOU NEED TO KNOW ABOUT NURSING

Nursing is a tremendous undertaking of time, dedication, and energy—more than either of you can possibly imagine. Your partner can spend eight hours (or more) in a twenty-four-hour day nursing. Nursing is a full-time job. It is also a practice and an art. While breastfeeding is natural, it does not necessarily follow that your partner will intuitively know how to do it. She needs instruction and support, as well as lots of fluids, good nutrition, and rest to successfully nurse.

Even though it may appear that a mother is just sitting and nursing, a nursing mother burns more calories and uses more energy than a man who works in construction. Give her this special time, to the best of your ability, without resentment or criticism. Your baby will flourish because of it. And the favor will be returned to you and your family a hundredfold.

It takes your partner and baby several weeks to become established in the art of nursing. Your partner may have times when she doubts her ability or desire to nurse. Your rock-solid confidence in her ability can support her through those times and make the difference between a successful, long-term nursing experience or a shortened, frustrated one.

Nursing is beneficial to mother and baby, and it helps the mother recover from birth. In order for your partner to have a *letdown* and release the milk from her breasts, her body must release the hormone *oxytocin*. Oxytocin helps the uterus contract back to its normal size and reduces postpartum bleeding, as well as engendering feelings of love in your partner. However, oxytocin cannot be released if your partner is anxious. Both mother and baby become fretful if your partner is having difficulty with her letdown.

If your partner is having trouble establishing nursing (and most first-time moms do), your calm, stable attendance can make the critical difference. Encourage her to seek help from a lactation specialist, La Leche League, a postpartum doula, or another experienced nursing woman. It takes about four weeks for a woman and her baby to establish the art of nursing; after that it becomes easier for both of them.

Your partner's body also releases the hormone *prolactin* when she nurses. Prolactin is referred to as the *mothering hormone*. It assists your partner in mothering the baby by calming and relaxing her so she can take greater joy in mothering. Nursing is one way body wisdom supports a woman to transition into her role as mother.

Nursing is also a way body wisdom protects the infant from disease. In the first several days, your baby is nourished by *colostrum*, which is a super-charged food designed for him. It is loaded with antibodies, provides a laxative that helps cleanse him of the sticky dark meconium stool, and coats the intestines to prevent harmful bacteria from attacking the digestive system. Colostrum nourishes your baby until mother's milk comes in.

It takes several days to a week for your partner's body to produce milk. Her breasts may get engorged when it comes in. This is uncomfortable for your partner, but once she has made it through, her milk supply adjusts to the needs of your baby, and keeps doing so periodically.

Sucking increases milk supply. As your baby grows, there will be times when he nurses more frequently. This is nature's way of increasing the supply for his changing needs. Nursing provides the skin-to-skin contact essential to the baby's physical and emotional development.

Human milk is also brain food. It supports the development of your baby's brain and nervous system like no other option. Sucking at the breast contributes to jaw, palate, and facial development. In addition, the protein and nutrients in mother's milk are easier for your baby to digest and assimilate than any other kind of milk.

Mother's milk supplies the infant with all the nutrition and fluids it needs for the first six months. The American Academy of Pediatrics recommends exclusive breastfeeding for the first six months. Your nursing baby doesn't even need additional water. Your partner's body is designed to grow, birth, and totally nourish the baby, and protect him from many illnesses. After six months, the baby requires food. Your partner may choose to nurse through toddlerhood (or beyond), and her milk will continue to supply your child with nutrition and antibodies, as well as the nurturing support he needs to grow into a healthy individual.

Whether your partner nurses several days, several months, or several years, your baby greatly benefits from nursing.

CAN YOUR PARTNER NURSE AND BOTTLE-FEED?

This option sounds like the best of both worlds. However, if your partner nurses, it is wise not to introduce bottles until nursing is well-established, which takes three to four weeks. When a baby sucks from a bottle, his mouth is positioned differently. Sucking from a bottle is also not as much work. If a baby gets too many bottles too early, he may reject the breast. However, if your partner chooses to bottle-feed, she might consider supplementing with occasional breastfeeding in the first week to offer her baby colostrum.

In the first several weeks, the mother's body is fine-tuning its milk supply. If a baby does not spend enough time sucking at the breast, the mother's body may not produce enough milk for the baby. Consequently, both mom and baby get frustrated which encourages bottle-feeding, which further reduces milk supply. And before you know it, the baby quits nursing.

Once mother and baby have firmly established nursing, an occasional bottle can be introduced without creating this downward cycle. Some women need to return to work and have to rely on bottles to feed the baby while they are gone. Many of them choose to rent a breast pump and freeze the milk. This approach keeps the milk supply established and gives the baby the highest-quality food while the mother needs to be away.

WHAT WOMEN SAY ABOUT NURSING

Isabelle, Miriam, and Emily, three of my postnatal yoga students, commented on their nursing experiences:

> *I remember sitting in the rocking chair with my baby, trying to get all the mechanics of learning how to nurse. And it's never what you imagine it's going to be. I had these huge breasts and this little tiny baby head down there. And you wonder, how does this all work? No wonder mother rhymes with smother. We have to watch it that we don't smother our babies with this huge offering of a breast we have to give them.*

> *Sometimes the baby goes three hours between nursing. Usually, I'm asleep when that happens. But sometimes the baby nurses every other hour. So it's an hour on and an hour off. Nurse the baby twenty min-*

utes on one side; change the baby's diapers; nurse twenty minutes on the other side. Burp the baby. And I've got an hour in that nursing session. Nursing is a full-time job and that's what I couldn't quite imagine.

Once I got the hang of it, nursing was really rewarding. I mean, when can someone so easily and totally satisfy the needs of another human being? All I had to do was sit there, nurse, and enjoy the baby.

WHAT MEN SAY ABOUT NURSING
Four fathers—Ethan, Jeremy, James, and Noah—related their observations and satisfaction regarding their partners' nursing experiences:

I couldn't have been a stronger advocate. I sort of had an artist's eye in it. I didn't have to have my own experience, but I could appreciate the aesthetic.

My wife nursed without any real problems. It was such a cozy time for our family. She did get engorged when the milk came in, but that was temporary.

My wife tired easily when she nursed, and I had to keep encouraging her to get more rest. She also needed some assistance in the beginning, and her nipples got sore, but other than that, it was great.

Nursing was such a positive experience that I can't think of a downside to it. It added to the warmth and completeness of the experience. I wouldn't have had it any other way.

SEX AFTER BABY

The first few weeks after birth, there is a fair amount of drainage, called *lochia,* which drains from the uterus as it returns to its normal size. If your partner has stitches from tears or an episiotomy, these need to heal completely before sex is resumed. Speak with your doctor or midwife; they often recommend a six-week sabbatical on sex after the birth. However, some medical caretakers suggest waiting only four weeks in individual situations. Your partner's individual healing and inclination also determine how soon you resume sex. Here are a few things you should know:

- Women may be too exhausted to think about sex for a while.
- A lot of men are exhausted too. Both men and women need time to recover and adjust after birth, because so many changes are occurring in their lives and in their relationships.
- Oral sex during the healing phase is not recommended because of the possibility of infection.
- Sometimes a woman gets touched-out by nursing and holding the baby, and cannot handle more touch until she has a chance to renew. Be patient.
- Women's estrogen levels are low during the recovery period and during full-time nursing, which influences sexual desire. Because of lowered estrogen, a woman may experience dryness and need to use a sexual lubricant.
- If a woman exclusively nurses, her estrogen levels are low enough to prevent ovulation. It is nature's way of preventing pregnancy. However, once additional bottles or food are given to the baby, a woman's estrogen level may spike enough for her to ovulate. Even if she has not yet had a menstrual period, a pregnancy can occur. Be sure to discuss contraception with one another and your medical caretaker.
- Many women discover that sex after birth is more pleasurable than sex before birth. Giving birth opens up awareness to sensation in the vagina, which can increase sexual pleasure.

SEXUAL LIBIDO, NURSING, AND FAMILY LIFE

A woman engaged in exclusive breastfeeding has lowered levels of estrogen and progesterone, which suppress ovulation, the menstrual cycle, fertility, and sexual libido. Once food from other sources is introduced, estrogen and progesterone levels rise, causing ovulation, fertility, and the menstrual cycle to resume. It is not abnormal for a woman who is predominantly nursing to have no menstrual cycle for as long as a year. Women who do not nurse generally ovulate around forty to forty-five days postpartum and their menses begin eight to fourteen days later.

Increased levels of prolactin during nursing, which compel a woman to mother, also decrease sexual libido. Though her sex drive is naturally suppressed, it does not interfere with her ability to have orgasm. Body wisdom alters female biochemistry. It also alters male biochemistry.

In studies done with animals, males who are closely involved with a female and her young have higher levels of vasopressin, which supports monogamy and fatherly behavior.[12] In addition, men who live with their partner and infant naturally produce higher levels of oxytocin, which engenders love for their partner and baby, reduces blood pressure, and may contribute to reducing future heart disease.[13] To concur with hormonal changes in their partner, men produce higher levels of prolactin, which tempers sexual desire, but not the ability to achieve orgasm.[14]

Men need to understand that women may not be inclined to initiate sex for many moons after birth. Don't take it personally. She may be willing, but she may need more touch and cuddling before you initiate sex. Because elevated prolactin levels contribute to relaxation, some women let-go and enjoy sex more after birth than they did before. Since you are both producing higher levels of oxytocin, which encourages bonding behavior, connect with her regularly through touch. Knowing the reasons behind the changes in your partner's sexual desire can help you relax and enjoy each other more during this transitional time.

FATHERHOOD IS A CALLING

Society does not acknowledge the rapid, immense growth men undergo as they take up their roles as fathers. Nor does it acknowledge the fact that one of the most self-developing acts a man takes is to answer the call of fathering and family life. To contemplate fatherhood is to realize that being a father defines and personifies the great spiritual teachings. As fathers, men learn and live the hardest and the highest spiritual practices: unconditional love, humility, generosity, discernment, joy, gratitude, honesty, compassion, patience, forgiveness, and service without expectation. Fatherhood is a fast-paced spiritual path.

Fathers practice these spiritual teachings, model them, and pass them onto their children. What you deposit into your child in the first several years takes up a short time in your life, but it is your child's whole life. Your child's developing character is deeply rooted in the first five years. These years are crucial because they are the foundation your child builds upon as he matures.

If a child receives unconditionally loving attention regularly from even one person in the first five years, his chances of navigating successfully through the challenges of life are greatly increased. Fathers cannot inoculate their children against life's calamities. But fathers can offer them attentive love, the single most powerful, undeviating, and directing force to guide them. Fathers can also offer the mother of their child love, respect, and support, which makes their child feel more secure, happy, and confident.

When fathers offer whatever love they have to give in the moment, they live with the freedom and satisfaction of knowing they showed up with what they had and gave it. In the ecology of the sacred, it is in receiving that we give. And it is in the very act of giving that we receive. From this perspective, offering does not diminish us; it increases us, and it increases others.

Answering the call of fathering does not mean fathers do not grapple with it or fall and fail in it from time to time. But it does mean when they honestly assess their lives, they know they gave what they had to give in the circumstances they were in at the time. They were there in the struggle of doing the work they were called to do, and they were committed to it.

To practice the art of fathering imperfectly, but with a sincere heart, is a more sane approach than being burdened by trying to follow an impossible script. As Phil, an experienced father of four, said: *They'll probably turn out all right in spite of my best intentions.* Gaining a perspective on what is important and what is not, gracefully accepting your very human oversights, finding humor in the situation, and being forgiving and patient with yourself as you navigate fatherhood is high-level practice.

Modeling discernment, acceptance, good-natured humor, patience, and forgiveness toward yourself and others in the midst of life's demands gives your child a map for how to live his life. You teach your child *how to be*, as well as *what to do*. This frees you and your child from the burden of having to do everything right, and it gives you more capacity to witness and accept the unique, individual person your child is. This is a great gift to your child.

Deposit your love deep into your child, and your love will stay with him forever, even after you are gone. Your child will pass your love on to his child, and it will go from generation to generation.

THE BEGINNING

Your partner underwent tremendous physical and emotional changes and challenges through pregnancy and birth. But now, you and your partner will have your lives stretched and reshaped again. Once you and your partner have passed through the journey and challenge of labor and birth, you begin an even greater journey. You embark on an even more challenging and remarkable undertaking.

You will never have a relationship quite like the one you are about to have with your child. It will test your abilities and restructure your life. You will grow emotionally and spiritually. You will discover love like you have never known it. Our children are our teachers. They give us more than we give them. You will learn what only someone for whom you are willing to sacrifice your life for can teach you.

As Monty, an experienced father, said to Lars, a new father: *You have no idea what you are in for. And no one can tell you, because you wouldn't believe it. Hang on for the ride.* It is hard to imagine the amount of work and challenge your child will bring into your life. But it's also hard to imagine the amount of joy and satisfaction your child will give you. Enjoy your baby!

ENDNOTES

1   Rudolph Ballantine, MD, Radical Healing: Integrating the World's Great Therapeutic Traditions to Create a New Transformative Medicine (Three Rivers Press, 2000), 391.

2   Howard Kent, Breathe Better, Feel Better (Allentown: People's Medical Society, 1997), 82.

3   Kent, Breathe Better, Feel Better, 82.

4   Justin O'Brien, PhD, The Wellness Tree: The Dynamic Six-Step Program for Creating Optimal Wellness (Saint Paul: Yes International Publishers, 2000), 63.

5   Donna Farhi, The Breathing Book: Good Health and Vitality Through Essential Breath Work (New York: Holt Paperbacks, 1996), 9.

6   Kent, Breathe Better, Feel Better, 10.

7   Henci Goer, Obstetric Myths Versus Research Realities: A Guide to the Medical Literature (Westport: Bergin & Garvey Paperback, 1995), 252.

8   Pam England, CNM, MA, and Rob Horowitz, PhD, Birthing from Within: An Extra-Ordinary Guide to Childbirth Preparation (Albuquerque: Partera Press, 1998), 197.

9   Penny Simkin, PT, The Birth Partner: Everything You Need to Know to Help A Woman Through Childbirth, Second Edition (Boston: Harvard Common Press, 2001). (This is an excellent guide with good medical information.)

10 Janet Balaskas, Active Birth: The New Approach to Giving Birth Naturally, Revised Edition (Boston: Harvard Common Press, 1992), 15.

11 Anne Lamott, Grace (Eventually): Thoughts on Faith (New York: Riverhead Hardcover, 2007), 180.

12 Natalie Angier, "What Makes a Parent Put Up With It All?" New York Times, February, 28, 2008.

13 Linda F. Palmer, DC, "The Chemistry of Attachment," Attachment Parenting International News, Vol. 5, No. 2, 2002.

14 Angier, "What Makes a Parent Put Up With It All?".

APPENDIX 1

OPTIONS TO DISCUSS WITH
THE PRACTITIONER BEFORE BIRTH

DURING PREGNANCY:

- Find a skilled practitioner you and your partner are confident in and comfortable with. It is wise to attend some of your partner's prenatal checkups to give you an opportunity to get to know the practitioner before birth.

- Discuss your practitioner's view of intravenous fluids (IVs) and electronic fetal monitors (EFM). If you and your partner prefer to avoid their use, discuss the option of having these waived. However, give your practitioner the freedom to use medical judgment, if their use is warranted. Inquire if a wireless monitor is available.

- Discuss the practitioner's practices on episiotomies. You want a practitioner who does not routinely perform episiotomies, who supports the perineum after the baby crowns, and who allows the baby's head to emerge at its own pace. However, give your practitioner the freedom to use medical judgment if an episiotomy is warranted to facilitate birth. You and your partner may want to request that no episiotomy be performed, unless there is a medical reason that warrants one.

- Discuss what pain medication options your practitioner prefers to use. Inquire about the benefits and disadvantages. If your partner prefers to use pain medication, she may want it administered as soon as possible after arriving at the facility. Let your practitioner know. If you and your partner prefer to avoid medication, let your practitioner know. Also let your practitioner know you prefer an internal exam be performed to avoid pain medication being administered once your partner is in transition labor (eight to ten centimeters dilated).

- Would you like to catch the baby? If so, give your practitioner a heads up.

- Would you like to cut your baby's cord? Let your practitioner know.
- Do you want the baby's cord blood stored? Do you want to donate it? Do you want the placenta? If so, discuss these options with your practitioner.
- Let your practitioner know that you and your partner would like as much time as possible with your baby after birth to give you both bonding time before the baby is weighed, measured, and undergoes its medical routine. Of course, if there is an emergency, the health of mom and baby is primary.

APPENDIX 2

REVIEW OF LABOR TERMS (CHAPTER 8)

TERMS TO KNOW

- **Effacement** is thinning of the cervix.
- **Dilatation** is opening of the cervix. The cervix must be dilated to ten centimeters and 100 percent effaced before pushing begins.
- A **mucus plug** forms along the length of the cervix during pregnancy and is sometimes released with a **bloody show** during labor.
- The **placenta** is a large disc-shaped, meaty organ attached to the inside wall of the uterus. Its function is to provide the baby with nourishment and oxygen and remove wastes.
- The baby is attached to the placenta by its **umbilical cord.** Oxygen and nourishment travel from the placenta through the umbilical cord to the baby. The baby's wastes also travel through the umbilical cord to the placenta for removal.
- The baby and the umbilical cord are surrounded by the fluid-filled **amniotic sac** (bag of waters) for protection.
- **Braxton-Hicks** contractions tone the uterus; they do not efface or dilate the cervix.
- **Prelabor** contractions may occur during late pregnancy. They begin the process of dilating and effacing the cervix.
- **Internal exams** are performed periodically during pregnancy and labor to determine the effacement and dilation of the cervix. Dilation measurement is not an accurate gauge of when labor will begin or how long labor will last. Don't put too much emphasis on the dilation measurement.
- Once labor begins, **time contractions.** Time a series of five consecutive contractions periodically to determine the frequency and length of contractions. Intensity of the contractions is determined by observing your partner's behavior.

- The purpose of **intravenous fluid (IV)** is to keep the woman's body hydrated during labor. IVs are also used to administer some drugs, if needed. The purpose of the **electronic fetal monitor (EFM)** is to track and record the baby's heart rate, as well as the frequency, duration, and intensity of the contractions. Neither is needed for a woman whose labor is progressing normally; however, they are often used routinely in hospital births.
- If the back of the baby's head is facing the mother's belly, this position is called **anterior occiput.** Anterior position is optimal for mother and baby. A baby in anterior position initially presents facedown as it emerges out of the birth canal.
- About 25 percent of the time, the back of the baby's head is facing the mother's back. This position is called **posterior occiput.** A mother whose baby is in posterior position experiences more back pressure and usually needs firm counterpressure on her lower back. A baby in posterior positions presents faceup as it emerges out of the birth canal.
- An **episiotomy** is a surgical incision that increases the diameter of the vaginal opening to accommodate the birth of the baby's head. In many births, episiotomies are unnecessary.

APPENDIX 3

REVIEW OF STAGES OF LABOR (CHAPTER 9)

THREE STAGES OF LABOR:
- **Stage I: Dilation**—This stage is divided into three phases: Early, Active, and Transition. The purpose of the first stage is to completely efface and dilate the cervix to ten centimeters so the baby can move out of the womb and into the birth canal. During the dilation stage, dramatic changes occur. Your partner changes from a person you know into a woman totally absorbed and taken over by labor. Early labor is generally manageable, but active labor demands your partner's entire energy.
- **Stage II: Pushing and Birth**—The purpose of the second stage of labor is birth. This is the pushing phase, also known as the descent stage. The baby descends out of the womb, through the birth canal, and is born. This is a dynamic stage. Your partner comes out of the consuming labor trance and becomes more alert. She focuses her energy to do this one most important and holy work—birth the baby.
- **Stage III: Delivery of the Placenta**—The purpose of the third stage is to deliver the placenta, also called the placental stage. The placenta is referred to as the afterbirth. During this stage, you and your partner will be entranced by your new baby and relieved that labor is behind you. Hold your baby during this period and immerse yourself in the experience.
- A normal labor lasts anywhere from two to twenty-four hours (or more). An average first time labor lasts twelve to seventeen hours.

APPENDIX 4

CHECKLIST FOR THE BIRTHING ROOM (CHAPTER 19)

WHAT TO DO WHEN YOU ARRIVE AT THE BIRTH FACILITY

- Help your partner get physically comfortable in her new surroundings. She may want to sit in a rocking chair, squat, get on her hands and knees, or lie on the bed in side-lying position. Make sure her position is aligned and supported. She may also need time alone in the bathroom.
- Once your partner is comfortable, make another trip to the car, if needed, to get whatever you may have left behind.
- Locate the small, semi-circular vomit pan (or bags) in the bedside table. Place on top of the table. If she vomits, it will be within easy reach.
- Locate the cabinet in the room with extra towels, wash cloths, and blankets. You may need to request extra blankets to use to support your partner's alignment, as well as for warmth.
- Request an extra pillow or two. Use them to support your partner's alignment during labor. (Combine the blanket and pillow request).
- Locate the dirty linen container. You will throw washcloths and towels in it after bathing, showering, etc.
- Provide or request fluids for you both.
- Request a birthing ball. It's easy to roll around and use in any space. When your partner is not using the ball, you can sit on it and be close to her. You can also stretch your back over it to relieve some tension.
- Be courteous to the staff. Thank them for their assistance. A little courtesy goes a long way.
- Dim the lights. Play music. (Most rooms are equipped with portable CD players.)
- Cut distractions and make the environment conducive to the process of labor.

TEND YOURSELF
- Place your packed bag in a convenient location.
- Do your three-step, one-minute-centering practice to gauge and refine your alignment, breath, and focus.
- Focus your attention on your partner.

IF LABOR IS PROGRESSING RAPIDLY, DO THE MOST IMPORTANT
- Help your partner into a comfortable, supported position.
- Get fluids for you both.
- Get out the vomit pan (or bags).
- Dim the lights.
- Do your centering practice to prepare yourself to be the mountain and the warrior.

APPENDIX 5

ESSENTIAL TIPS FOR LABOR

YOUR THREE MAIN GOALS
- Be the mountain—maintain your stability.
- Be the warrior—be responsive to your partner's cues and protect her space.
- Be centered—use the three-step, sone-minute centering practice over and over again to maintain your vigil.

FOUR WAYS EASY WAYS TO CARE FOR YOUR PARNTER
- Keep her warm. If she gets hot, offer a cool washcloth or ice pack.
- Offer sips of water regularly.
- Help her change positions regularly.
- Observe her alignment and help keep her comfortable—support head, torso, lower back, hips, knees, and feet, when appropriate

FOUR POINTERS FOR COMMUNICATION
- Talk to her within a twelve inch radius of her face.
- Touch and talk to her from your center.
- Minimize questions, instructions, and distractions, especially during contractions.
- Use running-interference technique to be a go-between for communication, when appropriate.

FOUR WAYS TO TEND YOURSELF
- Use breath awareness, the one-minute centering practice, and soft gazing to relax.
- If you lose it, dive into your breathing.
- If your partner tethers you in a hand grip, offer her handgrips to secure her hands.

- Drink fluids and eat or drink a protein supplement, if you get hungry.

TAKE HER TO THE BATHROOM REGULARLY (CHAPTER 21)

- Take her to the bathroom every hour—with a fifteen to thirty minute leeway.
- Do not give her a warning. After a contraction is over say: *It's time to go to the bathroom.* Then, immediately help her get up.
- If she has an IV, make sure the IV line is free. Unhook the EFM (if she is using one).
- If she has a contraction on the way to the bathroom, stop and do slow dancing.
- Turn the water on in the bathroom and leave it running until she urinates.
- Take your cue from your partner whether to leave her in privacy or stay with her.
- If you stay with her, let her lean your body into yours for support.
- Give her as much time as she wants. Bathroom position is great for mom and baby.

APPENDIX 6

STRATEGIES TO HELP MANAGE PAIN (CHAPTERS 10, 11, &13)

INTERVENTION STRATEGIES
- Use simple breath awareness and be aware of your own breath, as well as your partner's.
- Use a nasal decongestant spray, if needed, to keep her nasal passages open.
- If her breath becomes erratic, rapid, shallow, or exhibits long pauses, use hand-on-upper-abdomen technique.
- Use sounding technique with the aaahhhhh sound. This sound helps to keep her mouth soft and her jaw unclenched.
- Keep the pitch of her voice low. Use a low-toned sound near her ear.
- Monitor facial tension with a touch-and-say.
- Do labor one wave, one breath at a time.
- Use 5-to-1 countdown technique to help your partner through a hot-spot of accelerating labor. Do several rounds in a row, if needed.
- Encourage a shower or bath. Water promotes relaxation and pain relief.
- Help her to change positions regularly.
- Use hot packs. You can also use cold and hot packs alternately.
- If nothing works, use breathe-in-breathe-out technique at the tip of her nose.

USE FOCAL POINTS AND MOVEMENT RITUALS
- In early labor, suggest using the cervix as a focal point. She breathes in and out through the cervix while she visualizes opening.

- Encourage her to use dive-into-pressure technique. She takes her awareness right to the pressure and breathes into it and through it to soften and release.
- Go to the beach technique. She keeps her mind focused at the diaphragm and lets the waves of labor wash over and through her.
- Use a chosen word like, soften, or a phrase that works for your partner.
- Encourage a movement ritual like rocking or stroking.
- Use touch, massage, or press on pressure points in the hands or feet, etc.

BETWEEN WAVES: HELP HER RELAX

- Encourage her to release tension from the previous wave with a sighing exhalation, when needed.
- Help her establish flowing breath at the diaphragm by using hand-on-abdomen.
- Use a touch-and-say to relax and soften eyes, jaw, mouth (one focus at a time).

USE WISDOM WHEN DECIDING ON MEDICATION

- If your partner chooses to use medication for pain relief before the onset of labor, support her 100 percent. She may want drugs administered as soon as possible after arriving at the birth facility.
- If your partner chooses to avoid drug use, but requests them during labor, use the pain relief skills listed above before the staff administers pain medication.
- Request an internal exam before administering pain medication.
- Once your partner is in transition labor (eight to ten centimeters dilated), pain medication may be problematic because it decreases sensation for pushing.
- If she uses drugs, her mobility will be restricted. Get her up to use the bathroom before a drug is administered.

APPENDIX 7

FREQUENTLY USED LABOR POSITIONS (CHAPTER 16)
- Walking
- Supported standing
- Slow dancing position
- Supported back stretch
- Rocking in a rocking chair—support head, lower back, and feet, when appropriate.
- Sitting on a ball—combine with light bouncing, pelvic tilting, side-to-side rocking, or pelvic circling.
- Tailor sitting
- Squatting and supported squat positions
- Frog position
- All-fours and supported all-fours positions
- Side-lying position—observe alignment and support head, legs, and feet.
- Be creative with positions.

APPENDIX 8

HOW TO ASSIST YOUR PARTNER
IF LABOR STALLS (CHAPTER 20)

IF LABOR STALLS

- Suggest a bathroom trip. Remain with her and help support her position. Or if she prefers, shut the door and give her privacy for as long as she wants.
- Make sure she is warm.
- Offer fluids.
- Suggest a walk. Keep the conversation light and see if you can make her laugh.
- Help her establish flowing breath. Use hand-on-abdomen technique.
- Encourage her to relax her face. Use a touch-and-say. If the face is relaxed, the whole body relaxes and relaxation can facilitate labor.
- She may enjoy sitting in tailor position while she talks with you and connects. She can also combine this position with cervix breathing.
- Squatting may assist the baby to move into a more optimal position which may help progress. Once she is comfortable in her chosen squat position, encourage her to establish a deep, slow, rhythmic breath. Suggest she combine the breath with tension and release of the pelvic floor. Once your partner has united the breath with the tension and release of the pelvic floor, she becomes centered, calm, and focused which may help labor continue.
- Sitting on the ball to bounce, rock, circle, or do pelvic tilts may help the baby to move into a more optimal position. She can combine movement with the breath to increase her focus.
- An all fours or frog position is a good position for lower back discomfort. You can provide counterpressure and she can

combine it with pelvic tilting and tension and release of the pelvic floor with the breath.

- If labor stalls in early labor, a shower is preferable to a bath because standing uses gravity. Go into the shower with her and do slow dancing or leave her alone to give her privacy, whichever she prefers. If labor stalls after several hours, she may prefer a bath because she may be exhausted and need to rest.
- If labor stalls because of exhaustion, first make a bathroom trip and offer fluids. Then tuck her into bed. Give her body lots of support, make sure she is comfortable, turn out the lights, and let her rest. You need to rest too. If the bed is large enough, crawl into bed with her. Allow your breath to become fluid and flowing. As your body relaxes, it will help your partner relax.
- If you are in a hospital, your medical attendant may recommend pitocin. If you and your partner want to hold off on using medication be sure to inquire whether there is a reason you can't wait before administering pitocin.
- Resist the urge to fix it. Don't instruct your partner. Let her find her own way. Remain calm. Most of the time labor spontaneously begins on its own.
- Remain confident. The baby will come.

APPENDIX 9

PUSHING REVIEW (CHAPTER 24)

QUICK TIPS TO ASSIST YOUR PARTNER DURING PUSHING
- Help your partner into a comfortable pushing position. Most common are the semi-sitting and squat positions.
- Remind her to take a full breath and release the breath in intermittent, grunting spurts.
- Remind her to use all three diaphragms and the abdominals to regulate and increase power.
- Remind her to press deep, low, and out.
- Use a touch-and-say to release facial tension.
- Encourage her to let body wisdom do its work instead of using sheer willpower.
- Use opposition (push-pull technique) to increase opening and make her pushing more effective.
- Between contractions encourage her to use fluid diaphragmatic breathing, soften the face, and rest. Change positions, when appropriate.

INDEX

Note: Page numbers shown in **bold** include images relevant to the associated term.

INDEX

THE ST. JOHN BIRTHING METHOD:

HOW TO GET MORE INFORMATION

The concepts, practices, techniques, and strategies presented throughout *Fathers at Birth: Your Role in Bringing Your Child into the World* are part of the St. John Birthing Method™. Practical and conceptual, the St. John Birthing Method™ offers an integrated view that deals with the human and transcendent aspects of birth. Based on medical science, sound yogic principles, and the author's methods developed and proven during years of practice, this method provides couples with the knowledge, skills, and tools they need to have the most rewarding birth experience possible.

Fathers at Birth is derived the St. John Birthing Method™ and is written for the father-to-be to who wants a clear understanding of his role during labor, birth, and the early days of fathering. It specifically addresses the man who wants to know what his laboring woman needs from him, how to meet those needs, and how to transform himself into a confident and responsive birth companion. It also answers the need of the woman who wants her man to know how to be the best birth companion possible. When a man understands his vital role during the birthing process, both men and women benefit significantly.

Mothers at Birth by Rose St. John, the companion book to *Fathers at Birth*, is scheduled to be released by Ringing Bell Press in 2009. Also based on the St. John Birthing Method™, it addresses pregnancy, birthing, nursing, and the early days of mothering with the same straightforward and practical, yet conceptual and transcendent approach. For information on *Mothers at Birth*, go to ringingbellpress.com.

To get more information about *Fathers at Birth* and to receive a complimentary MP3 relaxation download, go to fathersatbirth.com.

To request a speaking or training event by Rose St. John contact publicist@ringingbellpress.com.